Cradle to Grave

Studies in the History of Medicine

Edited by Charles Webster, All Souls College, Oxford

Volume 4

PETER LANG

Oxford · Bern · Berlin · Bruxelles · Frankfurt a.M. · New York · Wien

Alysa Levene, Martin Powell, John Stewart
and Becky Taylor

Cradle to Grave

Municipal Medicine in Interwar England and Wales

PETER LANG
Oxford · Bern · Berlin · Bruxelles · Frankfurt a.M. · New York · Wien

Bibliographic information published by Die Deutsche Nationalbibliothek.
Die Deutsche Nationalbibliothek lists this publication in the Deutsche Nationalbibliografie; detailed bibliographic data is available on the Internet at http://dnb.d-nb.de.

A catalogue record for this book is available from the British Library.

Library of Congress Cataloging-in-Publication Data:

Cradle to grave : municipal medicine in inter-war England and Wales / Alysa Levene ... [et al.].
p. ; cm. – (Studies in the history of medicine ; v. 4)
Includes bibliographical references and index.
ISBN 978-3-03910-904-3 (alk. paper)
1. Public health–England–History–20th century. 2. Public health–Wales–History–20th century. 3. Social medicine–England–History–20th century. 4. Social medicine–Wales–History–20th century. I. Levene, Alysa, 1976- II. Series: Studies in the history of medicine ; v. 4.
[DNLM: 1. Public Health–history–England. 2. Public Health–history–Wales. 3. History, 20th Century–England. 4. History, 20th Century–Wales. 5. Local Government–history–England. 6. Local Government–history–Wales. 7. Social Welfare–history–England. 8. Social Welfare–history–Wales. 9. State Medicine–history–England. 10. State Medicine–history–Wales. WA 11 FA1]
RA487.C73 2011
362.10942‘09041–dc22

2011005811

ISSN 1424-7933
ISBN 978-3-03910-904-3

Hochfeldstrasse 32, CH-3012 Bern, Switzerland
info@peterlang.com, www.peterlang.com, www.peterlang.net

Contents

Preface and Acknowledgements

The origins of this volume lie in the early 2000s. Martin Powell and John Stewart (then at the University of Bath and Oxford Brookes University respectively) had been working separately on aspects of inter-war health care. On the basis of this complementarity of interests they submitted a bid to the Wellcome Trust for a three year Project Grant to support a research programme on municipal medicine in inter-war England and Wales. The essence of this proposal was that public sector health care of the 1920s and 1930s had been little researched and was, in consequence, not properly understood. The bid was successful and our first acknowledgement is therefore to the Wellcome Trust.

The grant allowed for the employment of Alysa Levene and Becky Taylor as Research Officers and between them they tackled both quantitative and qualitative aspects of the project. The immediate outcomes of this work were four co-authored articles in the *Bulletin of the History of Medicine*; *Urban History*; *Medical History*; and *English Historical Review* (see Bibliography for full references). Some of the material found in the present volume derives in part from these journal articles and we gratefully acknowledge the support of the respective editors and anonymous referees, not least for comments which were uniformly helpful and constructive. Papers deriving from our research were given at a wide variety of locations and again we are grateful to those participants who provided feedback on our work.

Archival and library research necessarily incurs many debts, both professional and personal. We would like to thank the staff of the local record offices in Lewes, Barnsley, Cwmbran, and Middlesbrough; of The National Archives; of the Bodleian Library, University of Oxford and the Official Publications Room, University of Cambridge; and Councillor Michael Stokes who both granted access to Barnsley Labour Party archive and gave up time to be interviewed. Becky Taylor would also like to personally thank Glen Rangwala, Ben Rogaly, Kirat Randhawa, Alex, Gareth, Seren and Brambles Housing Co-op for accommodation and friendship during archival visits; and Rossport Solidarity Camp which hosted much of the writing of the West Hartlepool and Newport chapters. Further financial support was received from the Oxford Brookes Centre for Health, Medicine and Society: Past and Present, and the Centre for the Social History of Health and Healthcare, a collaborative venture between Glasgow Caledonian and Strathclyde Universities at Glasgow Caledonian University. We owe a great debt to Dr Richard Biddle for his careful work with the typescript.

Finally, we wish to acknowledge the patience of the Peter Lang staff (like many academic endeavours this volume is somewhat overdue); and Professor Charles Webster, not only in his capacity as series editor but also as a scholar whose own work sets the standard for the proper understanding of health care in twentieth century Britain.

Abbreviations

BALS	Barnsley Archives and Local Studies
BMA	British Medical Association
ENT	Ear Nose and Throat
ESRO	East Sussex Record Office
GCRO	Gwent County Record Office
GP	General Practitioner
MCW	Maternity and child welfare
MO	Medical Officer
MOH	Medical Officer of Health
MP	Member of Parliament
NHS	National Health Service
PACs	Public Assistance Committees
PAI	Public Assistance Institutions
PEP	Political and Economic Planning
PHCs	Public Health Committees
SLA	Swansea Library Archives
SMA	Socialist Medical Association
TB	Tuberculosis
TNA	The National Archives
VD	Venereal disease
YMA	Yorkshire Miners' Association

List of Tables and Figures

Tables

Figures

CHAPTER ONE

Introduction

The British 'cradle to grave' William Beveridge welfare state, much of which historically has been viewed as highly centralized, has the NHS as its centrepiece. After over sixty years of the NHS it is difficult to envisage a different health care system. However, those of the Nordic countries have at various points been based on local government and before 1948 local government provided the main quantitative backbone of health care in Britain as well.[1] Moreover, virtually all contemporary observers, including many civil servants at the Ministry of Health and leading national and local political figures, expected a future national health service to be based on local government, and Aneurin Bevan's bold stroke of nationalising health care was dismissed as impractical less than a decade before 1948.

In this book we aim to provide a reassessment of municipal medicine in interwar England and Wales.[2] In doing so, we take a wider view of municipal medicine than just the 'medical'; rather, we aim to situate the health services in the wider context of a local government system. This localist lens provides a salutary and usefully different perspective than that taken by many previous studies. A. J. P. Taylor opens his account of *English History 1914–1945* with his well known claim that 'until August 1914 a sensible, law-abiding Englishman could pass through life and hardly notice the existence of the state, beyond the post office and the policeman.'[3] However we argue that

1 T. Grønlie, 'Norwegian General Hospitals, 1970–2002: County Ownership – an Interlude Between Welfare Localism and State Direction', *Medical History*, 50:2 (2006), 189–208.

2 For Scotland and Ireland, see PEP, *Report on the British Social Services* (London, 1937).

3 A. J. P. Taylor, *English History 1914–1945* (Harmondsworth, 1970), 25.

this understates the importance of local government or the local state. As early as 1889 Sidney Webb indicated the importance of municipalism in everyday urban life with his vignette of the 'individualist town councillor' who unwittingly takes in the benefits of more than a dozen municipal services – including the municipal hospital and lunatic asylum – on his way to prepare a speech on nationalisation.[4]

Harling also reports the 'modest sort of cradle-to-grave social provision' in a local historian's paean to Liverpool Corporation at the turn of the century:

> It offers to see that the child is brought safely into the world. It gives him playgrounds to amuse himself and baths to swim in. It sees that the citizen's house is properly built and sometimes even builds it for him. It brings into his rooms an unfailing supply of pure water from the remote hills. It guards his food and tries to secure that it is not dangerously adulterated. It sweeps the streets for him and disposes of the refuse of his house. It carries him swiftly to and from his work ... If he is sick it nurses him; if he is penniless it houses him; and when he dies, if none other will, it buries him.[5]

In the same vein John Davis reports a writer of 1900 claiming that 'food, shelter, education, work, leisure, wholesome amusement, a living wage, security against poverty, provision for old age, and all other necessities can be made certain for all by use of existing powers.'[6] Joseph Chamberlain made a similar remark of Birmingham in 1876, of his term as Lord Mayor between 1873 and 1876. During that time – he wrote – Birmingham was 'parked, paved, assized, marketed, Gas-and-Watered and improved – all as a result of three years active work.'[7] This was still true of Birmingham in the early twentieth century, when Neville Chamberlain entered the

4 Quoted in D. Fraser, *The Evolution of the British Welfare State* (3rd edn, Basingstoke, 2003), 122.

5 P. Harling, *The Modern British State: An Historical Introduction* (Cambridge, 2001), 123.

6 J. Davis, 'Central Government and the Towns' in M. Daunton ed., *The Cambridge Urban History of Britain*, iii: *1840–1950* (Cambridge, 2000), 284.

7 R. Self, *Neville Chamberlain. A Biography* (Aldershot, 2006), 19.

council, and in November 1928, during the second reading of his Local Government Bill, he stated that:

> [l]ocal government comes so much nearer to the homes, and therefore to the hearts of the people, than any national government can. ... They regard it as standing as a guardian angel between them and ill-health or injustice, and they look upon it, too, as something ... of a benefactor and a teacher in want ... I have seen for myself what local government can do, what I think it ought to do.[8]

According to the PEP 1937 Report on the British Social Services, '[n]ever before have the public services of the state been so continuously and intimately bound up with the family life of ordinary citizens as they have in recent years.'[9]

As these testimonies make clear, although the title of this book calls on a phrase generally linked with the post-1945 welfare state, it is one which can also be applied to the earlier era of municipally based politics. Mr Marshall, Labour MP and a former Lord Mayor of Sheffield stated that 'In one way or another, local government touches our lives at all stages from the cradle to the grave.'[10]

Focusing on Municipal Medicine

We have said that we take a broader view of municipal medicine in this book than many studies so far. Nonetheless, the definition of the term is problematic. Our definition operates within two limits. First, we examine 'medicine' largely in terms of personal health services.[11] This means that

8 Self, *Neville Chamberlain*, 19, 126; K. Feiling, *The Life of Neville Chamberlain* (Hamden, Conn, 1970, first published 1946), 52.

9 PEP, *Report on the British Social Services* (London, 1937), 10.

10 Hansard, House of Commons, 15 February 1945, col. 459.

11 See N. Wilson, *Public Health Services* (London, 1938); N. Wilson, *Municipal Health Services* (London, 1946).

we focus on personal/ individual and mainly curative health care rather than environmental/ sanitary services that aim to promote health in a wider sense.[12] Inevitably some services are dealt with in greater detail than others, but all tables and figures cover this remit unless indicated otherwise. Second, and more straightforwardly, we focus on 'municipal' rather than 'voluntary' provision. In essence this means health services funded by local government via ratepayer contributions (although this was often supplemented with grants from central government), as opposed to the voluntary services which were funded by a range of charitable and contributory schemes. These two sectors ran alongside each other but were quite different in origin and history, and often catered for different types of people. In fact, as Sally Sheard has pointed out, it is more accurate to speak of a trichotomy of healthcare provision rather than a dichotomy, with the third player being the poor law medical services.[13] Thus our focus on the municipal sector highlights one part of this triad only, although we are concerned in the later chapters of this book to set them in the wider context of healthcare provision. Indeed, when examining the workings of healthcare provision *locally*, it frequently becomes clear that the division between sectors was not so clear-cut to either users or providers as it is to later scholars.

At a macro level, however, this focus makes particular sense when we consider the separate providers of these different strands of healthcare. Our focus is on multi-purpose elected local government in the form of the County Boroughs in England and Wales. While there are problems of defining local government, we focus on the 'modern' system created in the 1880s and 1890s, and in particular on its top tier; the local authorities with the greatest powers of provision. This puts our spotlight predominately on ratepayers rather than paupers, who were served severally by

12 The discussion of local case studies in Chapters 4–7, however, indicate how far 'personal health' was still seen as part of a larger whole which included the environment, housing and infrastructure.

13 S. Sheard, 'Reluctant Providers? The Politics and Ideology of Municipal Hospital Finance 1870–1914' in M. Gorsky and S. Sheard, eds, *Financing Medicine: The British Experience Since 1750* (London, 2006).

the Poor Law Boards of Guardians, and the voluntary sector at the start of our period, although this changed to some degree over the course of our period, as we will show. Defined in this way, municipal medicine has a briefer time span than voluntary provision and the Poor Law, covering the period 1888–1948. Our focus is on the latter end of this period, for reasons we will go on to outline.

Despite its significance as a healthcare provider, however, municipal medicine has been neglected in the literature in terms of focus, scale and time. First, the main foci of attention have been directed at other sectors. As Robert Pinker puts it, the local authority hospital service – the most high profile, if by no means only form of municipal medicine – went unpublicised as it engendered 'neither the loyalties of the voluntary movement nor the antipathies of the poor law.'[14] For example, there are many 'hospital histories' for former voluntary hospitals, but very few for former municipal hospitals. This probably at least partly reflects a desire to focus on 'cutting edge' surgery and innovations at the top of the medical hierarchy, which is where the voluntary hospitals tended to specialise. Less attention has been paid to the 'less interesting' and less high profile areas such as chronic medicine – where the municipal and poor law sectors played an overwhelmingly prominent role. This has contributed to the view that the municipal sector was inferior to the voluntary. Social policy accounts also tend to be gloomy, with the partial exception of Harris, who still ultimately reaches rather pessimistic conclusions.[15] Welfare historians have been eager to embrace the idea of a 'mixed economy' of providers, but while Gray regards

14 R. Pinker, *English Hospital Statistics 1861–1938* (London, 1966), 79.

15 For example, see E. Midwinter, *The Development of Social Welfare in Britain* (Buckingham, 1994); P. Thane, *Foundations of the Welfare State* (2nd edn, Harlow, 1996); K. Jones, *The Making of Social Policy in Britain: From the Poor Law to New Labour* (London, 2000); N. Timmins, *The Five Giants* (London, 2001); G. Peden, *British Economic and Social Policy: Lloyd George to Margaret Thatcher* (2nd edn, Hemel Hempstead, 1991), xii; D. Gladstone, *The Twentieth-Century Welfare State* (Basingstoke, 1999); B. Harris, *The Origins of the British Welfare State: Society, State and Social Welfare in England and Wales, 1800–1945* (Basingstoke, 2004); M. Bruce, *The Coming of the Welfare State* (4th edn, London, 1968).

the health service sector in the interwar period as composed of a similar 'mixed economy of health care', medical historians– like contemporary patients– have been wary of entering the municipal sector.[16]

Second, in terms of scale, there has been a similar polar focus on the national aggregate data, or local studies of individual areas, hospitals and services. For example, John Welshman has focused on Leicester and Barry Doyle on Middlesborough, while John Pickstone deals with the sector in England's north-west. Other local studies take in areas such as Coventry, Bristol and Sheffield [17] Particular services have been dealt with by, for example, Brian Abel-Smith on hospitals, Linda Bryder and Francis Smith on TB, and Lara Marks and Jane Lewis on MCW, while biographies focus on key individuals like Neville Chamberlain and Aneurin Bevan.[18] While these

16 A. Gray, 'A Mixed Economy of Health Care: Britain's Health Service Sector in the Inter-War Period' in A. McGuire, P. Fenn and K. Mayhew, eds, *Providing Health Care: The Economics of Alternative Systems of Finance and Delivery* (Oxford, 1991). G. Finlayson, *Citizen, State, and Social Welfare in Britain, 1830–1990* (Oxford, 1994) and J. Stewart, 'The Mixed Economy of Welfare in Historical Context' in M. Powell, ed., *Understanding the Mixed Economy of Welfare* (Bristol, 2007) on the mixed economy, and for the reluctance to open this view to the municipal sector, M. Powell, 'What was Wales? Towards a Contextual Approach to Medical History' in P. Michael and C. Webster, eds, *Health and Society in Twentieth-Century Wales* (Cardiff, 2007).

17 J. Welshman, *Municipal Medicine: Public Health in Twentieth Century Britain* (Bern, 2000); B. Doyle, 'Competition and Cooperation in Hospital Provision in Middlesbrough, 1918–1948', *Medical History*, 51:3 (2007), 337–56; J. Pickstone, *Medicine and Industrial Society: A History of Hospital Development in Manchester and its Region, 1752–1946* (Manchester, 1985). Further, our own work has engendered further research in the area – see, for example J. Neville, 'Explaining Variations in Municipal Hospital Provision in the 1930s: A Study of Councils in the Far South West', PhD thesis, University of Exeter, 2010.

18 B. Abel-Smith, *The Hospitals 1800–1948* (London, 1964); L. Bryder, *Below the Magic Mountain: A Social History of Tuberculosis in Twentieth-Century Britain* (Oxford, 1988); F. B. Smith, *The Retreat of Tuberculosis 1850–1950* (London, 1988); L. Marks, *Metropolitan Maternity: Maternal and Infant Welfare in Early-Twentieth Century London* (Amsterdam and Atlanta 1996); J. Lewis, *The Politics of Motherhood: Child and Maternal Welfare in England, 1900–1939* (London, 1980); Feiling, *The Life of*

studies provide important pieces in the jigsaw, a more holistic overview is still lacking. There has not been a comprehensive treatment of the sector in Britain since the work of Norman Wilson.[19] While we have information on national trends in particular services, and on the broader picture for local case studies, there has been little 'middle range' work that places areas in their national context.[20] Given the large variations that characterised municipal provision, we argue that a contextual view is vital.[21]

Third, turning to the temporal dimension, the interwar period has been overlooked in comparison with the period of Poor Law medicine (from the 1860s up to 1928) and the post-1948 NHS.[22] It is notable that more general historical works neglect municipal medicine in interwar Britain, for example, the number of people dealt with by the sector notwithstanding.[23] This was, nonetheless, a crucial period in the evolution of British state medicine not least because of the impact of the vital but historiographically neglected 1929 Local Government Act. This abolished the Poor Law Unions and Guardians, and transferred their services to the municipal sector. In doing so, it enabled local authorities in England and Wales to take over Poor Law institutions to be developed as general hospitals. Like much local government legislation, this Act was permissive in character. In other words, this 'external shock' had very different impacts in different parts of the country. This means that national figures hide large geographical variation, making local studies which are placed within a broader national context all the more vital.

Neville Chamberlain; D. Dilks, *Neville Chamberlain*, i: *Pioneering and Reform, 1869–1929* (Cambridge, 1984); Self, *Neville Chamberlain*.

19 Wilson, *Public Health Services*; Wilson, *Municipal Health Services*. Welshman's *Municipal Medicine* is largely a study of Leicester.

20 For national trends, see Pinker, *English Hospital Statistics*. For examples of local case studies see note 15.

21 Powell, 'What was Wales?'.

22 Thane also notes the neglect of the period 1918–48 (*Foundations of the Welfare State*, xiii).

23 For example, R. Overy, *The Morbid Age: Britain Between the Wars* (London, 2009); and M. Pugh, *'We Danced All Night': A Social History of Britain Between the Wars* (London, 2008).

For all of these reasons, it is important to turn our attention back to the municipal sector and the interwar period. While municipal medicine did have significant problems of coverage and equity, we attempt to present a more nuanced picture in a broader context. In particular, we aim to explore three key questions: first, how did patterns of expenditure on municipal medicine vary in aggregate and also disaggregated by service, over space and over time? Second, what factors explained these national and local patterns? And third, to what extent are these observations confirmed by a purposive sample of four local case study areas? These questions are addressed in turn in the chapters which follow. Before that, we will use the remainder of this chapter to explain further the development and shape of the municipal medical sector.

The Evolution of Municipal Medicine

To outline the evolution of the municipal medical sector, it is necessary to start with those that preceded it: the voluntary and poor law services. Put simply, the various institutions and charities within the voluntary sector – of which the voluntary hospitals are the best known – were founded to cater for the 'deserving poor' through the philanthropy of the rich. They came in all shapes and sizes: large and small, general and specialist, but tended to exclude the chronic sick and those with infectious disease. These gaps produced a patchy service, albeit one which at its best performed its functions very well, and by the mid-1930s the state was stepping in to plug some of these areas of 'voluntary failure'.[24] The problems of voluntarism were recognized by the sector itself, resulting in enquiries such as the 1919 Sankey Commission and the resulting attempt at coordination. These can be seen as direct responses, moreover, to the 'success' of the

24 M. Gorsky, and J. Mohan, 'London's Voluntary Hospitals in the Interwar Period', *Nonprofit and Voluntary Sector Quarterly* 30:2 (2001).

municipal sector in at least some areas of the country and the aggressively anti-voluntary hospital stance of certain parts of the Labour movement, which although unsuccessful at national level in the 1930s was much more so at local level. This was especially true for the 'flagship' local authority, the London County Council.[25]

On the other side were the poor law medical services. These were co-ordinated by the local Board of Guardians, and were originally intended for sick. They have been seen, albeit rather contentiously, as the 'origins of the NHS'.[26] It is generally claimed that these services improved in the late nineteenth century, with moves in some cities from sick wards in the mixed infirmary to separate Poor Law Infirmaries. Gradually staffing and equipment improved, and the client group widened beyond the pauper class. As early as 1905 the Poor Law provision had been termed the 'real hospitals of the land'. However, in many rural areas, provision was still largely in sick wards in the general workhouse that prompted parallels with Dickensian images of corruption and squalor. In London, however, the Metropolitan Asylums Boards had built up a vast empire that has been termed 'England's first state hospitals' that catered for the destitute sick, including mental illness, infectious disease and chronic sickness.[27]

Outside London, provision for infectious disease was the responsibility of Sanitary Authorities rather than the Poor Law Unions, although many Sanitary Authorities made arrangements with Poor Law authorities. Public Health Acts of 1866 and 1875 provided the power to erect 'hospitals or temporary places for the reception of the sick' although this was generally confined to cases of infectious diseases. Under Section 132 of 1875 Public Health Act paupers could be treated in municipal hospitals and the costs recovered from the Poor Law authorities. For non-paupers (in principle) the individuals were liable for the cost. While local authorities had technically had the power to provide general hospital services for

25 J. Stewart, *The Battle for Health: A Political History of the Socialist Medical Association, 1930–51* (Aldershot, 1999).

26 R. Hodgkinson, *The Origins of the National Health Service* (London, 1967).

27 G. Ayers, *England's First State Hospitals 1867–1930* (London, 1971).

their non-pauper populations since 1875, therefore, only three authorities (Bradford in West Yorkshire; Willesden in West London; and Barry in South Wales) exercised that power before the 1920s.[28]

From this point on it is possible to trace a gradual accruing of powers to provide health services by the local authorities. The newly created County Councils of 1888 were given some role in the treatment of infectious disease by Acts of 1889, 1893 and 1901. From 1894 sanitary administration was reorganised into County Boroughs and into urban and rural districts.[29] Although private predated public provision for TB, by 1910 there were about 800 beds in thirty-two private sanitoria compared to over 2700 beds in seventy-eight public sanitoria.[30] Under the 1921 Public Health (Tuberculosis) Act, the County Boroughs and country councils in England and Wales became responsible for TB prevention and treatment. However, the small size of population and financial capacity meant that provision for infectious disease was often the responsibility of 'Joint Boards' of constituent areas, an arrangement which will be important for the local case study part of our investigation.[31]

The 1929 Local Government Act is usually taken as the point of departure for accounts of municipal involvement in general hospital provision. As has already been noted, this key change swept away the Poor Law Guardians, and transferred their facilities to the major local authorities of County Boroughs and County Councils.[32] The old functions of the Poor Law were

28 J. Mohan, *Planning, Markets and Hospitals* (London, 2002); PEP, *Report on the British Social Services*, 77.

29 J. Eyler, 'Scarlet Fever and Confinement: The Edwardian Debate over Isolation Hospitals', *Bulletin of the History of Medicine*, 61 (1987); Sheard, 'Reluctant Providers?'.

30 M. Worboys, 'The Sanatorium Treatment for Consumption in Britain 1890–1914' in J. Pickstone ed., *Medical Innovations in Historical Perspective* (Basingstoke, 1992),; Smith, *The Retreat of Tuberculosis*; Bryder, *Below the Magic Mountain*.

31 W. Robson, *The Development of Local Government* (rev. edn, London, 1948).

32 Abel-Smith, *The Hospitals*; J. P. Bradbury, 'The 1929 Local Government Act: The Formulation and Implementation of Poor Law (Health Care) and Exchequer Grants Reform for England and Wales (Outside London)', PhD thesis, University of Bristol, 1991; M. Powell, 'An Expanding Service: Municipal Acute Medicine in the 1930s', *Twentieth Century British History*, 8:3 (1997). The Act also brought a change to the

given in the first instance to PACs of the major local authorities. However, councils were encouraged to provide services through functional rather than client-based mechanisms, enabling in the words of the Webbs and the 1909 Minority Report of the Royal Commission on the Poor Laws the 'break up of the poor law'. In the case of medical services, this meant that the PHCs could unify facilities by operating them through their Public Health rather than PACs. In particular, they could take over, or 'appropriate' workhouse buildings or infirmaries for use as municipal general hospital.[33] This might appear to be of only minor terminological importance, but it carried great symbolic significance as it effectively granted greater rights of citizenship to paupers who had previously been disenfranchised by seeking relief.[34] It also has the potential to significantly expand the existing municipal health facilities for the bulk of the population. A political as well as a medical or administrative project, the intention was to reduce stigma in the use of services and allow councils to plan across the whole field of medical services. It was only after 1929 that the former poor law and infectious disease strands could fuse together into a more unified service.

---

grants system, from percentage matching grants, to a 'block grant' which was related to the borough's social and economic needs. It also contained several clauses regarding changes to the rating system. For more detail see Wilson, *Municipal Health Services*, 148–9; D. N. Chester, *Central and Local Government; Financial and Administrative Relations* (London, 1951), 288–9.

33 Local authorities had technically had the power to provide general hospital services for their non-pauper populations since 1875, but only three authorities had done so before the 1920s. The 1929 Local Government Act is therefore usually taken as the point of departure for accounts of municipal involvement in general hospital provision. Crowther states that the 1929 Local Government Act saw the creation of a 'hospital system which relied neither on charity nor on the Poor Law.' (M. A. Crowther, *British Social Policy* (Basingstoke, 1988), p. 73). See also Sheard, 'Reluctant Providers?'; T. Willis, 'The Bradford Municipal Hospital Experiment of 1920' in M. Gorsky and S. Sheard, eds, *Financing Medicine: The British Experience Since 1750* (London, 2006); Mohan, *Planning, Markets and Hospitals*, 37.

34 Crowther claims that the Local Government Act was one of the most important pieces of legislation of the twentieth century, while W. M. Fraser terms it 'one of the important landmarks in the history of Public Health' (Crowther, *British Social Policy*, 47); W. M. Frazer, *A History of English Public Health, 1834–1939* (London, 1950), 261.

However, although the powers of the Poor Law Unions had been transferred to the municipal sector, responsibility for some services was still divided between different local authorities, resulting in a confusing division of responsibilities.[35] Moreover, the water was muddied by the fact that the 1921 Tuberculosis Act had already made local authorities responsible for non-pauper cases, although they were encouraged to treat all cases. In the 1920s many TB patients were still accommodated in Poor Law infirmaries. Birmingham claimed to be only local authority in the country that treated all cases under its TB scheme in 1925. By contrast in South Shields all TB patients were accommodated in the Poor Law infirmary. In spite of the revolutionary potential of the 1929 Act, there were still over 3000 TB patients in PAIs in 1938.[36] A further strand of the 1929 Act was that councils must consult with the voluntary hospitals before planning any changes to provision. This, in principle, allowed a greater integration between public and private sectors, although this again relied on local take-up.[37]

The interwar period, then, saw an evolution from largely separate systems, with limited contact between them, towards a more diffuse pattern. As the 1944 White Paper put it:

> in earlier years the two systems had little working contact with each other and each went its own way with its own kind of service to the public. In recent years, however, there has been an increasing tendency for the two systems to get closer together, to realise their common aims in the service of the public and the value of a greater degree of organised partnership in improving that service together.[38]

Although there was no longer a *de jure* division of labour, *de facto* differences still existed.

35 Robson, *The Development of Local Government*.

36 Bryder, *Below the Magic Mountain*.

37 M. Gorsky, 'The Gloucestershire Extension of Medical Services Scheme: an Experiment in the Integration of Health Services in Britain before the NHS', *Medical History*, 50:4 (2006).

38 Ministry of Health, *A National Health Service*, Cd.6502 (London: HMSO, 1944), 55.

The Significance of Municipal Medicine

Sheard points out that provision can be measured in a number of ways.[39] Most research to date has used the number of beds in a hospital as an indicator of service, as this information is relatively easy to obtain. However, she argues that bed provision is only a useful proxy in the absence of better data, and suggests that expenditure is a better variable. Our approach supports this wider view since it is clear that hospitals were not the only indicator of a diverse or responsive healthcare service. Regardless of the exact measure, however, it can be shown that municipal medicine was an important and expanding sector that reached its apex in the 1930s before the Second World War and subsequent incorporation into the NHS. Indeed, municipal medicine was the quantitative backbone of the English healthcare offering, although its contribution varied by service. This is demonstrable even on the most simple measures: number of institutions, expenditure, staffing, beds, and patients treated.[40]

The precise contribution of municipal medicine towards health care overall is difficult to establish, however, as it varies according to different criteria and by different estimates. Webster writes that estimates of health expenditure for the 1930s differ, but according to Gray their 'broad consistency is reassuring'.[41] Much of the focus here has been on hospitals, although we stress again that any accurate view of the municipal sector must be broader than this. By way of indicative comparison, however, the figures put forward by historians indicate that publicly funded hospital services accounted for around 30 per cent and the voluntary hospitals for approximately 12 per cent of *total* expenditure. The remainder was accounted for by National Health Insurance and out of pocket expenses such as doctors'

39 Sheard, 'Reluctant Providers?', 119.

40 Powell, 'An Expanding Service'.

41 C. Webster, *The Health Services since the War*, i: *Problems of Health Care – The National Health Service before 1957* (London, 1988), 13; Gray, 'A Mixed Economy of Healthcare', 234–5.

and dentists' fees and self-medication. A number of estimates give municipal beds as a proportion of total beds in the 1930s.[42] Although precise figures differ, it is generally agreed that municipal hospitals accounted for about two thirds of all non-psychiatric beds.[43] However, the figures are very sensitive to strict definition. The proportions are very different if psychiatric beds are included or sick wards are excluded, for example.

Staying with the hospital example, it is also clear that aggregate figures hide a great deal of variation even within one sector. Here, disaggregated figures reveal an extremely varied division by type of bed. Pinker presents data from 1938 which shows that while the municipal sector did not have any of the country's teaching hospitals (although the Hammersmith Hospital was a Postgraduate Centre), it did house 54 per cent of general beds, 64 per cent of maternity beds, 27 per cent of other specialist beds and 91 per cent of beds for cases of TB, infectious disease and chronic conditions.[44] However, Pinker appears to have classified beds by hospital, and this disguises the fact that a general hospital may have had a mix of different types of beds. Nevertheless, this does not change the main conclusion that voluntary hospitals tended to pick (or cream-skim) their patients, leaving the municipal hospitals and the Poor Law medical service to care for those that remained. The Ministry of Health pointed out in 1944 that practically all chronic and less interesting cases were referred to municipal hospitals.[45] As Harry Eckstein puts it, municipal hospitals were seen as 'nothing more

42 *The Lancet* 28 October 1939, 946; Ministry of Health, *A National Health Service*, 41; Sir F. Menzies, 'Postwar British Medicine', *Medical Care*, 2:4 (1942); PEP, *Medical Care for Citizens*, Planning Broadsheet 222 (London, 1944).

43 See R. Titmuss, *Problems of Social Policy* (London, 1950), 66; M. Whitehead, *National Health Success* (London, 1988); Gray, 'A Mixed Economy of Healthcare'. Municipal beds formed 74 per cent of all beds in 1891, 78 per cent in 1911, 75 per cent in 1921 and 67 per cent in 1938. The annual growth rates for beds show that the faster rate for public (3.1 per cent) compared to voluntary beds (1.9 per cent) for the period 1891–1911 was reversed for 1911–21 (2.7 per cent voluntary and 1.1 per cent municipal), and for 1921–38 (2.6 per cent voluntary and 0.1 per cent municipal). See Pinker, *English Hospital Statistics*, 48–51.

44 Pinker, *English Hospital Statistics*.

45 Ministry of Health, *A National Health Service*, 43.

than the dumping grounds for the expensive chaff of the voluntary system.'[46] J. Rogers Hollingsworth argues that even though the differences between the public and voluntary hospitals were narrowing over time, there was considerable persistence in the differences between the two systems in their types of patients.[47] However, in London and other large cities, the municipal hospitals also treated acute cases, and we will go on to demonstrate that in some cases this translated into a first-class service. This shift is supported by Sir Fredrick Menzies' speculation that 'it is not an exaggeration to state that if war had not broken out in 1939, within another five years the best of the municipal hospitals would have equalled, if not indeed excelled, the best of the voluntary hospitals in all such vital matters such as buildings, equipment, staff and conditions of service.'[48]

Certainly the concentration of hospital beds had moved towards the municipal sector by the end of the interwar period. For example, the proportion of all non-psychiatric beds in local authority hands was 17 per cent in 1911, 23 per cent in 1921 and 47 per cent by 1938, mainly attributable to transfers following the 1929 Local Government Act. It should be noted that local authorities were also the principal providers of services for psychiatric provision. PEP's 1937 report on the British health services estimated that this sector housed 143,000 asylum beds and over 20,000 beds for mental defectives. Other estimates place this figure even higher.[49] By 1938, then, local authorities were the foremost providers of hospital services. PEP's 1938 report on hospitals stated that the local authorities provided about 62 per cent of total bed accommodation in Great Britain, quite apart from mental patients and mental defectives. They also reiterated that the sector provided almost all of the beds for infectious disease cases and chronic cases, as well as a hefty proportion of the country's institutional provision for

46 H. Eckstein, *The English Health Service: its Origins, Structure and Achievements* (Cambridge, Mass, 1958), 67.

47 J. R. Hollingsworth, *A Political Economy of Medicine: Great Britain and the United States* (Baltimore, 1986), 28.

48 Menzies, 'Postwar British Medicine', 340.

49 PEP, *Report on the British Health Services* (London: 1937), 275–9; Webster, *The Health Services since the War*, i: *Problems of Health Care*, 9–10.

maternity and TB care.[50] Moreover, there had been a qualitative change in provision, with the sector (for example) providing many more outpatient services than they had a decade or two earlier, although still not as much as the voluntary hospitals. The same trend is true of surgical care, technical support and specialisation.[51]

One of the few pieces of quantitative evidence that compares activity between sectors comes from the 1939 Plan for British Hospitals.[52] According to the Lancet's 'Special Commissioner' Stephen Taylor, although municipal hospitals had so many more beds than the voluntary sector, their turnover of inpatients (751,277) was under two-thirds (compared with 1,145,433 in the voluntary sector). Furthermore, as already noted, the volume of out-patient work done by the voluntary hospitals was 'enormously greater'. Similarly, the 1944 White Paper claimed that the larger voluntary hospitals 'have developed into centres of medical learning and research. They have always been and are still leading in the treatment of acute and surgical cases and out-patients.'[53] However, in other areas the municipal hospitals were the principal providers, most prominently in general and chronic medical work.

We have dwelt on the hospital example here in order to illustrate some of the key differences between the sectors providing healthcare in the interwar period, and also some of the problems in making comparisons

50 PEP, *The Hospital System* (London, 1936), 6. Similar trends and problems are identified for staffing levels, which is another indicator of development. Here, double-counting and different roles within sectors makes accurate comparison very difficult, as does the absence of any measure of quality. Meanwhile, it seems that the large growth in nursing provision over the period was disproportionately concentrated in municipal and poor law hospitals. See Titmuss, *Problems of Social Policy*; J. R. Hollingsworth, and E. J. Hollingsworth, 'Public Organizations: The Behaviour of Hospitals in England and Wales' in E. James ed., *The Nonprofit Sector in International Perspective* (Oxford, 1990); B. Abel-Smith, *A History of the Nursing Profession* (London, 1960); Gray; 'A Mixed Economy of Health Care'; F. Honigsbaum, *Health, Happiness and Security* (London, 1989).

51 Powell, 'An Expanding Service'. See also PEP, *The Hospital System*.

52 'A Plan for British Hospitals', *The Lancet*, 28 October 1939, 945–51.

53 Ministry of Health, *A National Health Service*.

between them. However, health care was much more than just hospitals, although these were clearly among the most prominent of its points of contact with the public. It also encompassed clinics and dispensaries, home-visiting schemes and milk depots, voucher schemes to subsidise food and supplies, and a range of specialist institutions for mental illness, TB, MCW, and infectious diseases. In sum, both in the hospital sector and more broadly, municipal medicine can be shown to be an important provider of personal health care, contributing a significant proportion of total expenditure, staffing and activity. However, we need to look at more than its quantitative importance. Its provision must also be judged in qualitative terms, and among the most important markers in this regard is its place in relation to the voluntary sector, and the poor law. The municipal sector provided the bulk of residual categories the voluntary sector did not wish to, or have space to, address, and this was exacerbated after it took over many of the medical functions of the poor law from 1929. This included provision for chronic and infectious diseases, including VD. However, as we will go on to show, this qualitative distinction between the sectors did vary geographically and chronologically and in some places did become more balanced over time.

Municipal Medicine and Local Government

Most medical history accounts focus on the 'medicine' of 'municipal medicine', but it was, in turn, an important part of the wider local government system. While municipal medicine does not feature heavily in histories of local government, it was nonetheless one of the most significant areas of local authority spending, and can give important information on issues such as democratic accountability and responsiveness. This is underlined for the interwar period, which is often seen as the high period of local government. While writers such as Simon Szreter locate its zenith in the late nineteenth century, most others look to the 1920s and 30s as its heyday.[54] We need, therefore, to think more carefully about the role of municipal medicine within a wider local political system.

Accounts of interwar health policy have presented both optimistic and pessimistic viewpoints. Charles Webster, for instance, who is the author of the official history of the NHS, at various times covers both angles. In 1990, he stressed the atrophy of municipalism arguing that interwar health policy was characterized by strict Treasury discipline; a minimum legislative response with maximum reliance on permissive powers; strict control of new services to give the impression of adequate response to need while actually providing services only on a token basis; and a failure to distribute services according to need. However, in 1988 he wrote that where permissive powers were applied to the utmost degree, where rate revenue was buoyant, and where the local MOH pressed modern developments, the standard of service bore comparison with later counterparts under the NHS.[55]

54 S. Szreter, 'A Central Role for Local Government? The Example of Late Victorian Britain', *History and Policy* [online journal] (2002). http://www.historyandpolicy.org/papers/policy-paper-01.html accessed 14 July 2009; H. J. Laski, I. Jennings, W. A. Robson, E. Halévy, *A Century of Municipal Progress* (London, 1935); M. Loughlin, M. David Gelfand, and K. Young, eds, *Half a Century of Municipal Decline, 1935–1985* (London, 1985). On the significance of the interwar period see, for example, J. Stevenson, *English Social History 1914–45* (Harmondworth, 1984), 309; R. Lee, 'Uneven Zenith: Towards a Geography of the High Period of Municipal Medicine in England and Wales', *Journal of Historical Geography*, 14 (1988); Pickstone, *Medicine and Industrial Society*, 6; J. M. Mackintosh, *Trends of Opinion about the Public Health, 1901–51* (London, 1953), 131.

55 Welshman, *Municipal Medicine*, 253–4, 264–5; A. Hardy, *Health and Medicine in Britain Since 1860* (Basingstoke, 2001), 109; J. Mohan, *Planning, Markets and Hospitals*, 37; Harris, *The Origins of the British Welfare State*; J. Stewart, '"The Finest Municipal Hospital Service in the World"?: Contemporary Perceptions of the London County Council's Hospital Provision, 1929–1939', *Urban History*, 32:2 (2005); C. Webster, 'Health, Welfare and Unemployment During the Depression', *Past and Present*, 109 (1985). See also M. Gorsky, 'Public Health in Interwar England and Wales: Did it Fail?' *Dynamis*, 28 (2008); M. Powell, 'An Expanding Service'; C. Webster, 'Conflict and Consensus: Explaining the British Health Service' *Twentieth Century British History* 1:2 (1990), 143.

The municipal sector of the interwar years has other critics. John M. Eyler, for example, argues that the period compares unfavourably with the years 1906–14. George Peden writes that the public health services remained as fragmentary in the 1930s as it was earlier, and that outside London and certain other areas little had been achieved ten years after the 1929 Local Government Act. Keith Laybourn claims that although there were also special facilities for infectious disease and the like, the total provision of hospital beds was low for the population and was not distributed in such a way as to effectively tackle the health problems of the nation as a whole. Some explanation may be found for these criticisms in a desire for a progressive narrative culminating in nationalisation in 1948.[56] Even supporters of the sector could not deny, however, that it had obvious limitations in this period, most notably its geographical variability.[57]

Contemporaries are prominent among the authors of the more optimistic accounts. Sir Fredrick Menzies, for example, pointed to the great expansion of public health services after 1929, and especially of municipal hospitals. William A. Robson also flagged up the hospital service as expanding in scope and reach, while being increasingly removed from the 'taint' of the Poor Law.[58] However, some historians have also pronounced favourably on the municipal sector of the interwar years, including those who, as already noted, deemed it the high point of municipalism. Writers like Pickstone, Anne Hardy and Jane Lewis have all pointed out the growth in certain municipal health sectors, like public health and maternal and

56 J. Eyler, *Sir Arthur Newsholme and State Medicine 1885–1935* (Cambridge, 1997), 387–8; Peden, *British Economic and Social History*, 109; Bradbury, 'The 1929 Local Government Act', 310; Davis, 'Central Government and the Towns', 282; Mohan, *Planning, Markets and Hospitals*, 56; K. Laybourn, *Britain on the Breadline: A Social and Political History of Britain 1918–1939* (Stroud, 1998), 77–8; Harris, *The Origins of the British Welfare State*, 242.

57 For example, see M. Powell, 'Hospital Provision before the NHS: Territorial Justice or Inverse Care Law?', *Journal of Social Policy*, 21:2 (1992); J. Mohan, 'Voluntarism, Municipalism and Welfare: The Geography of Hospital Utilization in England in 1938', *Transactions of the Institute of British Geographers*, 28 (2003).

58 Menzies, 'Postwar British medicine', 338–40; Robson, *The Development of Local Government*, 18.

child welfare.[59] Between 1918 and 1939 some twenty pieces of legislation enhancing or expanding local health authority services were passed, and the interwar years have been seen as a 'golden age' of public health. Douglas E. Ashford claims that '[a]ll this is not to detract from the momentous decision to nationalize medical care in 1948, but only to show that, compared to most countries, Britain had moved substantially toward public medical care thirty years before the law was passed'.[60] This movement was largely at a local level.

National and Local Welfare States

It has been claimed that the British welfare state is 'perhaps the most thoroughly nationalised of all welfare states'[61] The less cited portion of T. H. Marshall's famous account of citizenship is also concerned to trace the move from local to national welfare.[62] We need, however, to be clear about what is meant by such terms.[63] Martin Powell suggests three main criteria that distinguish national from local services.[64] First, a national service should include little autonomy and no democratic input at local levels. In contrast, a key characteristic of local government is that decisions should be made by local people through the local ballot box. The interaction of local

59 Pickstone, *Medicine and Industrial Society*, 6; Hardy, *Health and Medicine in Britain*, 85–6; J. Lewis, *What Price Community Medicine? The Philosophy, Practice and Politics of Public Health Since 1919* (Brighton, 1986), 15.

60 D. Ashford, *The Emergence of Welfare States* (Oxford, 1986), 165–6.

61 Ashford, *The Emergence of Welfare States*, 298.

62 T. H. Marshall, *Citizenship and Social Class* (London, 1950); D. Ashford, *The Emergence of Welfare States* (Oxford, 1986); A. de Swaan, *In Care of the State: Health Care, Education and Welfare in Europe and the USA in the Modern Era* (Cambridge, 1990).

63 But see E. Page, 'The Value of Local Autonomy', *Local Government Studies* 8:4 (1982); E. Page, *Localism and Centralism in Europe* (Oxford, 1991); Ashford, *The Emergence of Welfare States*, 122.

64 M. Powell, 'In What Sense a National Health Service?' *Public Policy and Administration* 13:3 (1998); M. Powell and G. Boyne, 'The Spatial Strategy of Equality and the Spatial Division of Welfare', *Social Policy and Administration* (2001).

political forces produces diversity: localism tolerates – even celebrates – diversity rather than the imposition of national uniformity.[65] Indeed, local autonomy is deemed more important than territorial justice.[66] In the words of one local government commentator, John Stewart, 'local government is the government of difference'.[67]

The second criterion concerns funding. In a purely localist service, with the complete absence of central grants, local areas would rely on their own resources: a scenario termed by Newton the 'grantless society'.[68] Such a situation would entail the territorial equivalent of 'to him that hath' in which richer areas would have access to more local resources and where no financial redistribution would take place between areas. In contrast to pure localism, in which localities are totally reliant on their own resources, in a national service the centre allocates money according to central criteria in an attempt to secure horizontal equity in funding at the national level. In terms of the interwar period, we see a shift in grant income, which has a bearing on this question. From 1929, grants were apportioned centrally, taking local needs and income into account. This might be thought to have reduced local control, but in fact, by not specifying that the block grant be spent on any particular service, the new system may have given a greater degree of discretion to local authorities. This contrasts with the previous system which awarded grants as a percentage of expenditure on specific services.[69]

65 For example, see W. A. Robson, 'Labour and Local Government', *Political Quarterly* 24:1 (1953).

66 See B. Davies, *Social Needs and Resources in Local Services: A Study of Variations in Standards of Provision of Personal Social Services Between Local Authority Areas* (London, 1968); K. Newton, 'Central Government Grants, Territorial Justice and Local Democracy in Post-War Britain' in D. Ashford, ed., *Financing Urban Government in the Welfare State* (London, 1980); Page, 'The Value'; G. A. Boyne and M. Powell, 'Territorial Justice and Thatcherism' *Environment and Planning C: Government and Policy* 11:1 (1993).

67 Page, 'The Value', 30.

68 Newton, 'Central Government Grants', 12.

69 E. Page and M. Goldsmith, 'Centre and Locality', in E. Page and M. Goldsmith, eds, *Central and Local Government Relations* (London: 1987); D. N. Chester, *Central and Local Government* (London, 1951); C. Foster, R. Jackman and M. Perlman, *Local*

Third, central control and funding should lead to provision which is equitable according to centrally determined standards. National social citizenship should mean that equal citizens receive equal treatment irrespective of factors such as location (as well as class, race and gender). The strategy of equality has a spatial component, with the aim of achieving territorial justice.[70] There should be horizontal equity in treatment: need should get identical response in different areas. In short, a national service should be based on national as opposed to local citizenship, funded 'from each according to their ability', delivered 'to each according to their need' at the national level. Geographical location should make no difference to contribution or benefit: two individuals of identical income should pay the same amount towards the service and two individuals in identical need should receive the same amount of benefit regardless of location. The aim of a truly national service would be to make geography irrelevant. It can be seen that in these terms health care has moved from a broadly local to a national service after 1948, with the creation of the *National* Health Service.

Municipal Medicine as a Local Welfare State

Before 1948 local or municipal health care was regarded by most commentators as the goal of progressive policy, with a national health service seen as not practical in political terms.[71] Indeed, Aneurin Bevan – the founder of the NHS – overturned both Labour Party policy and a broad bipartisan consensus on municipal health care when he introduced his scheme for a national service. A belief in local government in general and municipal medicine in particular was a major element in the policy of the Labour Party. Groups such as the early Fabians, the Independent Labour

---

Government Finance in a Unitary State (London, 1980); B. B. Gilbert, *British Social Policy 1914–1970* (London, 1970).

70 J. Le Grand, *The Strategy of Equality: Redistribution and the Social Services* (London, 1982); Davies, *Social Needs and Resources*; Powell and Boyne, 'The Spatial Strategy'.

71 For example, see Stewart, *The Battle for Health*.

Party and the SMA were all strong supporters of municipalism. Places like Bradford were regarded as strongholds of 'municipal socialism', with well developed local services. The London County Council, captured by Herbert Morrison's Labour Party in 1934, was the largest municipal hospital authority in the world, with its Health Committee chaired by SMA President Somerville Hastings.[72]

The policy of the Conservative/ National Government had a somewhat different basis, looking to 'partnership' between voluntary and municipal sectors. While the Conservative party saw a long term partnership, however, the Labour Party and some civil servants in the Ministry of Health tended to favour a policy of 'creeping municipalisation' in which seats on the governing bodies of voluntary hospitals would be given to local authorities in exchange for financial support, leading to eventual municipal capture.

As late as 1944, great tributes were paid to local authorities by speakers from all the main parties during the Debate on the Local Government White paper.[73] One Conservative MP, David Eccles, stated that 'what a tremendous task we set ourselves when we insist on using independent local government as the vehicle for the execution of a social policy which is national in scope ... [but it] may conflict with blue-printed efficiency and with the attainment of uniform standards. To reconcile those two apparent opposites of decentralization and efficiency is our task.'[74] The National Liberal Member, Stanley Holmes argued that '[i]f fundamental changes remove from the people the control of their own affairs ... whatever gain there might be in efficiency – and that is a debatable point – is discounted by other and more far reaching consequences.'[75] The Labour MP and SMA member Fred Messer pointed to two types of service. 'For

72 Willis, 'The Bradford Municipal Hospital Experiment'. On London, see J. Stewart, 'Socialist Proposals for Health Reform in Inter-War Britain: the Case of Somerville Hastings', *Medical History*, 39:3 (1995); J. Stewart, '"For a Healthy London": The Socialist Medical Association and the London County Council in the 1930s', *Medical History*, 41:4 (1997); J. Stewart, '"The Finest Municipal Hospital Service in the World"?'.

73 Hansard, House of Commons, Debate on Local Government, 15 Feb 1944.

74 Ibid. col 437.

75 Ibid. col 469.

the impersonal services such as electricity, I do not care who administers them so long as they can be carried into every house in the country. However, for human services such as education and health care to get efficiency it may be necessary to have a large unit, but if we do that there is a danger that the unit may be too far removed from the people ... Local administration of all these human services is better.'[76] As the White Paper on Local Government put it, 'members and officers of local authorities have shown themselves capable of shouldering with marked success varied and novel responsibilities. For this they have earned the gratitude of the nation, and there is no reason to doubt that they will prove equally capable of dealing with the problems of post-war reconstruction.'[77]

There was a general opposition to unelected, ad hoc bodies governing healthcare. Lord Latham, leader of the London County Council, reacted angrily to the idea of non-elected health boards in 1941: the 'Fifth Columnists against democracy are planning to steal the people's municipal hospitals.'[78] Labour Secretary of State for Scotland in the Coalition Government, Tom Johnston, attacked ad hoc health authorities as a 'system of continental dictatorships' inconsistent with the principles of representative government.[79] Reflecting the SMA's 'immutable belief' in local democracy, its President Somerville Hastings wrote in 1941 that '[a]bove all else, the hospitals after the war must be under the control of the elected representatives of the people through the Ministry of Health and the local authorities.'[80] Similarly, Labour's 1943 policy document, 'National Service for Health' insisted that 'wide powers must be left to local authorities; it is they who must be responsible for the detailed administration of the service.'[81]

Indeed, initial plans for the NHS from 1938 were based on various forms of municipalism, notably joint authorities. Local authorities played a major role in the 'Brown Plan' of 1941 and Sir Henry Willink's White

76 Ibid. cols 474–5, 506.

77 'Local Government during the Period of Reconstruction', 1944–5, Cmnd 6579, X, 1.

78 Cited in Stewart, *The Battle for Health*, 142.

79 Webster, *The Health Services Since the War*, i, 49.

80 S. Hastings, *The Hospital Services*, Fabian Research Series: 59 (London, 1941).

81 Labour Party, *National Service for Health* (London, 1943).

Paper, 'A National Health Service' of 1944. After the demise of the Brown plan, neither the 1944 White Paper nor the NHS Act planned to secure a unified service. The Society of Medical Officers of Health criticised the White Paper for splitting the service between local authorities and Joint Boards, stressing the problems of divided responsibility for clinical and preventive aspects of work in areas such as TB.[82] As PEP put it, 'a medical service in which local authorities play no part is unthinkable.'[83] In the King's Speech Debate in 1945, Morrison announced that Bevan intended to return to the 1944 White Paper. The 1945 Labour Party Conference agreed that 'no scheme is acceptable which does not ... give to the local authorities control over municipal hospitals and medical services on statutory Health Councils and Committees'.[84]

It is clear that a large weight of opinion was behind the delivery of health services at a local level well into the 1940s, and that this covered a wide range of services. A number of commentators stress the debate in Cabinet between Bevan and Morrison as to national versus local organisation. According to Michael Foot, Bevan's biggest battle – the most crucial in the whole fight for the Health Service, even though it was fought behind closed doors – occurred in the Cabinet.[85] Bevan unveiled his plan for a national service to the Cabinet in a paper dated 5 October 1945. Morrison led the defence on behalf of his beloved local authorities, putting up an alternative paper complimenting the Minister of Health for his 'brilliant and imaginative' scheme but denouncing it severely as an attack on local government for which the Government had no mandate. At a Cabinet meeting on 18 October, Morrison argued that Bevan's unelected boards 'would either be mere creatures of the Ministry or they would have to be

82 Society of Medical Officers of Health, *The White Paper on a National Health Service* (London, 1944).
83 PEP, *Medical Care for Citizens*, 16.
84 Hansard, House of Commons, Debate on King's Speech, 21 August 1945.
85 J. Campbell, *Nye Bevan and the Mirage of British Socialism* (London, 1987); M. Foot, *Aneurin Bevan. A Biography*. ii: *1945–1960* (London, 1975), 132; Webster, *The Health Services Since the War*.

given a dangerous freedom to pursue policies of their own at the expense of the Exchequer.'[86] Clement Attlee summed up in Bevan's favour.

Bevan argued for national (Parliamentary) rather than local accountability: boards 'will be and they must be the instruments of the Ministry ... The most sensitive instrument in this country for bringing about effective administration is the Question on the Order Paper of the House of Commons ... in a good many instances, the relationship between the citizen and his MP is more direct than the relationship between the citizen and his local authority.' He argued that 'by taking the hospitals from the local authority and putting them under the regional boards, large numbers of people will be enfranchised who are now disenfranchised from participation in local government.'[87] In one of his most famous statements, Bevan argued that 'When a bedpan is dropped on a hospital floor its noise should resound in the Palace of Westminster.'[88] However, Morrison claimed that it was possible to argue that

> almost every local government function, taken by itself, could be administered more efficiently in the technical sense under a national system, but if we wish local government to thrive we must consider the general effect on local government of each particular proposal. It would be disastrous if we allowed local government to languish by whittling away its most constructive and interesting functions.[89]

Once Cabinet agreement had been reached, the local authorities and Labour MPs quietly accepted this reversal of party policy although the London County Council and the SMA continued to level criticisms at what

86 TNA CAB 129/3, Memorandum by the Lord President of the Council, 12 October 1945.

87 Hansard, Standing Committee C on NHS Bill, 15 May 1946 (col 52).

88 Hansard, Standing Committee C on NHS Bill, 15 May 1946, col 77; S. Jenkins, *Accountable to None: The Tory Nationalization of Britain* (Harmondsworth, 1996), 65; see also Foot, *Aneurin Bevan*. ii, 192–3.

89 TNA CAB 129/3, A Memorandum by the Lord President of the Council, The Future of the Hospital Services, 12 October 1945.

they saw as an unnecessarily centralised system.[90] Bevan's decision to kick over the ballot box prompted surprisingly few problems for Labour MPs in the NHS debate.[91] The only Labour dog to bark was Frederick Messer who asked 'why this loss of faith in the elective principle? Why lose faith in what we believe to be democracy?'[92] The Conservatives instead saw their chance to become the defenders of localism: to support the man in the Town Hall as opposed to Labour's gentleman in Whitehall – as well as the defenders, on a point of principle, of the soon to be nationalised voluntary hospitals. Speakers such as Henry Willink, Richard Law and Sir Harold Webbe taunted the Labour Party in general and Herbert Morrison in particular about their part in the demise of local government. Sir Harold Webbe claimed that the NHS Act signed the 'death warrant of local government'.[93] He considered that the system of local government that followed the Local Government Act of 1929 allowed public health to be planned as a whole, which gave a complete interlocking of the preventive and curative medical services. The NHS would reopen the gap between preventive and curative public health, and take health back to a position which would be worse than before the 1930s.[94]

The Parliamentary and Cabinet discussions make clear how overtly political the debates over municipalism versus nationalisation were. Some commentators have noted that the loss of health care was a major loss of function to local government.[95] Local authorities certainly acquired other functions after 1945 and their overall expenditure increased.[96] However, the foundation of the NHS can easily be equated with a major downsizing

90 Stewart, *The Battle for Health*; Stewart, '"The Finest Municipal Hospital Service in the World"?'.

91 Hansard, House of Commons, 2nd Reading of NHS Bill, 30 April 1946.

92 Ibid.

93 Ibid. Col 274.

94 Ibid. Col 367.

95 For example, B. Doyle, 'The Changing Functions of Urban Government', in M. Daunton, ed., *The Cambridge Urban History of Britain*, iii: *1840–1950* (Cambridge, 2000).

96 For example, D. Wilson and C. Game, *Local Government in the United Kingdom* (Basingstoke, 2002).

of the role of local government. David Blunkett, a Labour front-bench Minister of the early twenty-first century, writing with author and commentator Keith Jackson, sees nationalisation of health as 'Labour's great mistake'. Blunkett and Jackson claim that the NHS, for all its sophistication and success, has never achieved the same combination of local accountability, sensitivity and innovation as local government services.[97] White argues that the NHS marked 'the greatest creation of quangos in British administrative history ... [marking] the true beginning of that withering away of local democracy recognised belatedly by the Royal Commission on Local Government in England in 1969.'[98] It called the loss of the hospitals 'a great misfortune' that ought to be reversed, but five years later, the remaining local authority health services were nationalised too. It is no exaggeration to talk of the immiseration of local government in its present state, with powers largely abdicated to Whitehall at the centre (the Attlee model) and to school governors, urban regeneration companies, housing associations and so on at the periphery (the Thatcher model).[99] The issue of the appropriate balance between centre and periphery within the NHS continues to be a major political issue, and we will return to this debate in our conclusion.[100]

97 D. Blunkett and K. Jackson, *Democracy in Crisis: The Town Halls Respond* (London, 1987), 55, 64.

98 J. White, 'From Herbert Morrison to Command and Control: The Decline of Local Democracy' *History and Policy* [online journal] (2004), < http://www.historyandpolicy.org/papers/policy-paper-18.html> (accessed 17 July 2009).

99 Ibid. See also J. White, 'From Herbert Morrison to Command and Control: the Decline of Local Democracy and its Effect on Public Services' *History Workshop; Journal* 59:1 (2005).

100 See R. Klein, *The New Politics of the NHS: From Creation to Reinvention* (4th edn, Oxford, 2001), 14.

Sources and Approach

The foregoing discussion has set out the general remit of this book, namely the interwar municipal medical sector, but with an eye to healthcare as part of a political system as well as a provider of medical services. In more specific terms, we analyse the geographical and temporal variations in the municipal health sector in this period in both quantitative and qualitative terms. We draw on both statistical data and national and local archival material.

Our focus is on County Boroughs – the largest of the units of local government and the ones exercising the fullest range of powers in respect of health (and other) services – they were characterised by the local government expert William Robson in the 1950s as 'the most enterprising type of council.'[101] They were highly urbanised 'islands' within the administrative Counties, mostly with populations over 75,000 (the exceptions, such as Canterbury, had often been awarded County Borough status through ancient charters).[102] In aggregate the population of the County Boroughs comprised a third of the national total in the interwar period.[103] The local government expert J. H. Warren noted, in the mid-1940s, that the large size and comprehensive powers of County Boroughs made them the best

101 Robson, *The Development of Local Government*, 269. This is not to underestimate the degree of energy displayed in many County Councils, which were the tier 'below' the County Boroughs. There was also not-infrequent collaboration between County Boroughs and other neighbouring authorities, as we note particularly in the discussion on hospitals in Chapter 3, and in the local case studies in Chapters 4–7. However, the County Boroughs form a coherent set of authorities with a recognisably wide remit, and it would be beyond the scope of this study to look beyond them. The workings of other types of local authorities would, however, repay further study.

102 The population threshold was raised to 75,000 from 50,000 by the Local Government (County Boroughs and Adjustments) Act of 1926. V. D. Lipman, 'The Development of Areas and Boundary Changes 1888–1939', in C. H. Wilson, ed., *Essays on local government* (Oxford, 1948), 42–3.

103 S. V. Ward, *The Geography of Interwar Britain: The State and Uneven Development* (London, 1988), 157.

authorities for implementing unified services, and the same qualities make them particularly valid arenas for discussing healthcare and the workings of local government: 'the organism [of the County Boroughs] has the highest degree of elasticity, resource, economy and responsiveness to public need; and that springs essentially from that concentration of many-sided activity under unified local control which is the characteristic of this – the most highly developed type of English Local Government administration'.[104]

However, the County Boroughs were not evenly distributed around the country, initially because of the requirement of the minimum population threshold and later because of opposition from the administrative counties at allowing their major urban areas to secede from the County administration into the County Borough system. Doncaster was thus the only city which was successfully 'promoted' to County Borough status during the whole interwar period, although the boundaries of many existing boroughs were extended.[105] The outcome of this suspension in County Borough charters was that there were few boroughs in the more rapidly economically developing areas of 'inner Britain' (largely around London – although the capital itself was administered separately and was not a County Borough), and an over-representation of the more economically depressed areas of 'outer Britain' (particularly the north of the country and south Wales).[106] The advantage of this lack of change to reflect changing economic circumstances, however, is that almost exactly the same units are being compared throughout the period under study.

The principal dataset for the national-level discussions of investment in municipal healthcare (in Chapter Two) is the series of Local Government Financial Statistics (Annual Local Taxation Returns up to 1930). These form an almost continuous run of financial information on local authority expenditure by service over the period. The disruption of the

104 J. H. Warren, *The English Local Government System* (London, 1946), 45–6.

105 Lipman ('The Development of Areas') states that between 1929 and 1937 the boundaries of 49 County Boroughs had been extended, transferring more than the entire population of Brighton, and more than twice the acreage of Birmingham to the County Boroughs.

106 Ward, *The Geography of Interwar Britain*, 157.

Second World War meant that the last peacetime report was published for the financial year 1936/7. Administrative delays also resulted in an abridged report in 1921/2. For the purposes of this part of the investigation, therefore, the 'interwar period' is confined to the years 1922/3 – 1936/7. This also has the unintended benefit of focusing on the peacetime health services by removing the effects of the immediate aftermath of World War One, the move to a wartime economy prior to 1939, and the tentative start of Ministry of Health planning to reorganise the health services. For the period 1922–37 data are available on the overall financial circumstances of all the eighty-three County Boroughs in England and Wales, as well as their expenditure on individual health services.[107] We utilise these data to explore patterns of expenditure by County Boroughs on healthcare over time, over space and between sectors.

We have chosen to focus on expenditure data for this part of the study because it carries a measure of quality as well as quantity. The financial returns were audited centrally, and grants were subject to central approval (especially up to 1929 when the percentage grants were replaced by a needs-sensitive block grant, but even after this stage sanction was needed for extraordinary loans). This minimises the chances that some boroughs spent too extravagantly, although it is likely that this did occur to some extent.[108] There is also some acceptance in the literature on spending decisions that 'input' measures such as expenditure are frequently more accessible than 'output' such as number of beds per hospital nurse, and are frequently taken as a proxy for policy outcomes.[109] Variations in local costs and standards of

107 At the beginning of the period there were 82 County Boroughs; Doncaster was given County Borough status in 1927, so raising the number to 83.

108 Liverpool, for example, was characterised by the Ministry of Health in 1932 in a survey of its health services as being overly extravagant in its expenditure on social services: 'In marked contrast to many other industrial towns there is nothing niggardly in its administration. It carries itself with the air of a merchant prince, thinking in terms of millions, and distributing largesse with a ready hand', TNA MH66/721, Survey Report, Liverpool. However, comments such as these are rare.

109 For example, K. Hoggart, *Economy, Polity and Urban Public Expenditure* (Aldershot and Vermont, 1989), ii. R. Millward uses expenditure data as part of a factor analysis which is designed to capture a measure of quality of provision, see: 'Local Government

efficiency may have bought different quality or quantity of care in different areas but, overall, expenditure may be taken as a somewhat crude but acceptable proxy for quality. What are more debatable are the reasons underlying high levels of expenditure, and this may mediate the relationship between expenditure and quality. Some boroughs may have had to spend highly because their health service had been very poor previously, or because health conditions were very poor. In these situations high expenditure might not result in a high quality service. Conversely, a borough with a high proportion of wealthy inhabitants and good health and sanitation facilities might have lower demands made on its health services, necessitating lower levels of expenditure. Some of these considerations will be explored further in the chapters which follow. Nonetheless, as Sheard has noted, expenditure data do provide an accurate reflection of operating costs, and they have been a popular choice for measuring the quality of local government provision in several fields.[110]

A further comment is necessary on the coverage of the financial data. This study focuses on what was returned as 'general expenditure', plus loan charges. The two were classed together in the returns as 'total expenditure'. Capital expenditure was also recorded, but it is generally not included in the analysis except where this is made clear. There were two reasons for this omission. One was that capital outlay was unlikely to be a yearly charge, unlike general and loan charge expenditure, but instead consists of 'one-off' spending on larger projects. This makes it more suitable for study when considering large-scale projects like hospitals. Secondly, there was very little statistical correlation between general and capital expenditure over boroughs in a single year.[111] While this is interesting in itself, and will

Expenditure in Britain, 1870–1914: an Economic Analysis', *University of Manchester: Working Papers in Economic and Social History*, 27.

110 Sheard, 'Reluctant Providers?'. Examples of studies using local authority expenditure data are those carried out by F. Bell and R. Millward, 'Public Health Expenditures and Mortality in England and Wales, 1870–1914' *Continuity and Change* 13 (1998), Millward, 'Local Government Expenditure'; Robert Millward and Frances Bell, 'Economic Factors in the Decline of Mortality in Late Nineteenth-Century Britain' *European Review of Economic History*, 2 (1998).

111 Correlation coefficients between the two series were 0.191 for 1922, -0.003 for 1928 and 0.142 for 1934, for example.

be commented on briefly, it supports the assertion that the two types of spending should not be conflated. A concentration on 'general' expenditure will permit us to investigate the year to year trends which future parts of the project will endeavour to explain, by considering social, political and health variables for each of the boroughs, and analysing their relationship with levels and patterns of spending.

A second source of data is the annual report on local government elections published in *The Times* newspaper. We have noted already that local government was part of a wider political agenda, and that the Labour Party in particular was at this stage a staunch supporter of localism. The election data are used to test this association, to examine whether Labour influence on the council correlated with higher levels of expenditure. We choose to focus on Labour in particular, partly because of their historically strong association with local government, and also because of their prioritisation in many areas of socially ameliorative health services. Webster, for example, writes that 'Labour local authorities worked steadily towards the establishment of comprehensive municipal health services.'[112] Labour-controlled Bradford provided more maternity beds than any other place in the country and developed their municipal hospital before the passing of the 1929 Local Government Act. However, so did Liberal Barry, and T. Willis points out that Labour were in power in Bradford only during November 1919 – November 1920, and the chair of Health Committee was held by Liberals. He stresses instead the importance of cross-party support, and of the MOH.[113] The extent of Labour's direct influence is therefore complex, but the party remains associated with spending on health services, and was also the most easily identifiable local bloc in this era before party politics was fully taken on board in local government. The influence of the local Labour parties is explored in Chapter Two, and taken up again in greater detail in Chapters Four and Six.

112 C. Webster, 'Labour and the Origins of the National Health Service' in N. Rupke, ed., *Science, Politics and the Public Good* (Basingstoke, 1988), 184–202, 198.

113 Willis, 'The Bradford Municipal Hospital Experiment'; Laybourn, *Britain on the Breadline*, 63–4.

In Chapter Three we move on to discuss some of the reasons behind the national expenditure patterns outlined in Chapter Two. Here, the primary data source is a detailed but underused set of surveys of healthcare carried out by the Ministry of Health in the aftermath of the 1929 Local Government Act.[114] They survive for the majority of boroughs, and consist of reports and associated correspondence on the quality of municipal health provision. They offer a real and detailed insight into the decision making processes in different places, contextualised by the character of the town, its other needs, priorities and constraints. These range from financial considerations to council bickering, and thus allow us to uncover a range of factors which affected the way that money was spent, and healthcare services developed (or sometimes, not).

These surveys and their correspondence form the backbone of the detailed case studies which form Chapters Four–Seven. These were selected to represent four 'types' identified in existing studies as having a large impact on patterns of investment: a rich, Labour town (Newport), a rich non-Labour town (Eastbourne), a poor, Labour town (Barnsley), and a poor non-Labour town (West Hartlepool). The selection was based on the data explored in Chapter Two, and in particular aims to test the connections between wealth and politics on spending – although, as we will show, the labels are not necessarily accurate for the whole interwar period. In fact, the case studies indicate that expenditure patterns observed in Chapter Two were rarely the result of fixed characteristics, but were instead mutated through a whole series including local personalities, competing demands, and central steers, to name but a few. All four case studies call on a range of local-level information as well as the Ministry surveys, including council minutes, local newspaper reports, and memoirs. Between them, the case studies illustrate the political nature of local decision making, although this meant much more than the overtly political in a modern party sense. The combination of national-level data and local micro-studies is one of the principal novelties of this study, and the one of which we are most proud.

114 This is the MH66 series held at The National Archives. The surveys for the Welsh County Boroughs are catalogued under MH96.

Together, the two strands of work show us a detailed picture of municipal healthcare in this period of robust local government. The study ends with a reflection on how they join together, and what this suggests about ongoing debates about the shape of the NHS.

CHAPTER TWO

Patterns of Investment in Healthcare

In this chapter we explore patterns of expenditure by County Boroughs on healthcare over time, across regions and between medical sectors. As outlined in Chapter One, County Boroughs were the only unit of local authority administration responsible for the full range of health services. This makes a comparison of spending patterns particularly revealing of priorities and decision making over the whole spectrum. The data utilised in this chapter are the Local Government Financial Statistics (up to 1930 called the Annual Local Taxation Returns) which form an almost continuous series of financial information on local authority expenditure by service over the period.[1] The disruption of the two World Wars truncates the series slightly, so our focus here is on the period of financial years 1922/3 to 1936/7.[2] For this period data are available on the overall financial circumstances of all the eighty-three County Boroughs in England and Wales, as well as their expenditure on individual services.[3] As

1 S. Sheard, 'Reluctant Providers? The Politics and Ideology of Municipal Hospital Finance 1870–1914', in M. Gorsky and S. Sheard, eds, *Financing British Medicine: The British Experience Since 1750* (London, 2006). Examples of studies using local authority expenditure data are those carried out by F. Bell and R. Millward, 'Public Health Expenditures and Mortality in England and Wales, 1870–1914', *Continuity and Change*, 13 (1998); Millward, 'Local Government Expenditure in Britain, 1870–1914: an Economic Analysis', *University of Manchester: Working Papers in Economic and Social History*, 27; R. Millward and F. Bell, 'Economic Factors in the Decline of Mortality in Late Nineteenth-Century Britain', *European Review of Economic History*, 2 (1998).

2 Administrative delays produced a truncated report in 1921/2, and no reports were published after 1936/7 until after the Second World War.

3 At the beginning of the period there were 82 County Boroughs; Doncaster was given County Borough status in 1927, so raising the number to 83.

stated in Chapter One, our focus on provision over time, over geographical space and between sectors has been chosen as a corrective to much of the conventional wisdom that tends to focus on the aggregate picture at one point in time. As our analysis shows, this disaggregation reveals wide variation in temporal, spatial and sub-sectoral patterns.

Variations Over Time

There are many reasons to expect that patterns of expenditure will not have been static over the whole interwar period: fluctuating economic fortunes at a national as well as a local level; changing priorities in medical services arising from legislation and local needs; and a lessening need for infectious disease provision, to name but three. The overall trend was of growth across the whole sphere of public health (including environmental services such as sewerage and refuse collection) of the order of 20 per cent per year, compared with 2.5 per cent growth for all rate fund expenditure.[4] In the 1930s, public health was the fastest growing sector in expenditure terms, taking up 18 per cent of the outlay from rate funds by 1937. The personal – as opposed to environmental – health services which are the focus of this study formed a growing part of the broad sphere of public health. Between 1930 and 1936 they grew from accounting for 28.3 to 33.3 per cent of the gross public health budget, and from 4.7 to 5.9 per cent of all rate fund expenditure.[5] This reflects the changing priorities within the health field, and underlines the significance of the focus on personal health services.

4 R. Lee, 'Uneven Zenith: Towards a Geography of the High Period of Municipal Medicine in England and Wales', *Journal of Historical Geography*, 14 (1988), 265.

5 M. Powell, 'Did Politics Matter? Municipal Health Expenditure in the 1930s', *Urban History*, 22:3 (1995), 363.

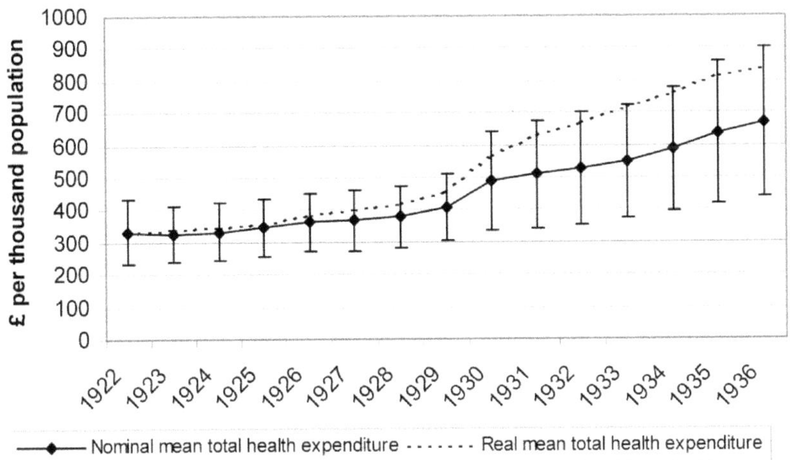

Figure 2.1 Mean County Borough Expenditure Per Thousand on Public Health, 1922/3–36/7

Source: Local Government Financial Statistics, 1922/3–36/7. Expenditure in real terms was calculated by applying relative changes in an index of retail prices to the expenditure on health. Price data from B. R. Mitchell, *British Historical Statistics* (Cambridge, 1988), Prices 10, Ministry of Labour/Department of Employment Indices of Retail Prices, UK, 1892–1980, pp. 739–41. The 'personal' public health services included are: mental deficiency, mental hospitals, infectious disease hospitals, general hospitals, tuberculosis services, maternity and child welfare, venereal disease services, notification of infectious diseases, miscellaneous health services, salaries of medical personnel, and vaccination.

The nominal and real trends (that is, adjusted for the cost of living) in spending on public health services over the period are shown in Figure 2.1.[6] Between 1922 and 1929, expenditure per thousand population increased very gradually. From 1929 there was a marked rise in spending on health, and the increased rate of growth continued for the rest of the period. This rise from 1929 was even more marked when deflation is taken into account, so that the increase was worth progressively more over the remainder of the

6 For details on the conversion to real spending see the note to Table 2.1.

period. The error bars illustrate the spread around the average expenditure over the dataset as a whole.[7] Their growing size indicates that the rise in aggregate spending was not spread evenly across all boroughs, producing a greater degree of overall variation from the mean (see below).

The principal factor behind the rise in expenditure in 1930 was the 1929 Local Government Act, which transferred spending on some of the poor law hospitals from the Poor Law Guardians' accounts (which were separate from the local authority administration) into the municipal Public Assistance and Public Health accounts.[8] They also promoted the unification of health services generally, prompting greater levels of investment at an aggregate level. The impact of hospital appropriation in particular is illustrated in Figure 2.2, which shows a much more gradual and uninterrupted upward trend once the spending on these institutions is removed. This points to the value of examining disaggregated expenditure if we are to make sense of overall patterns. While the trend in expenditure was still upward even when general hospitals are removed, it is their transfer into the public health remit which explains the dramatic upswing in the middle of the period. The nature of this transfer is described in greater detail in Chapter 3.

7 Each error bar indicates one standard deviation from the mean.

8 See Chapters One and Three for more on the mechanism behind this transfer.

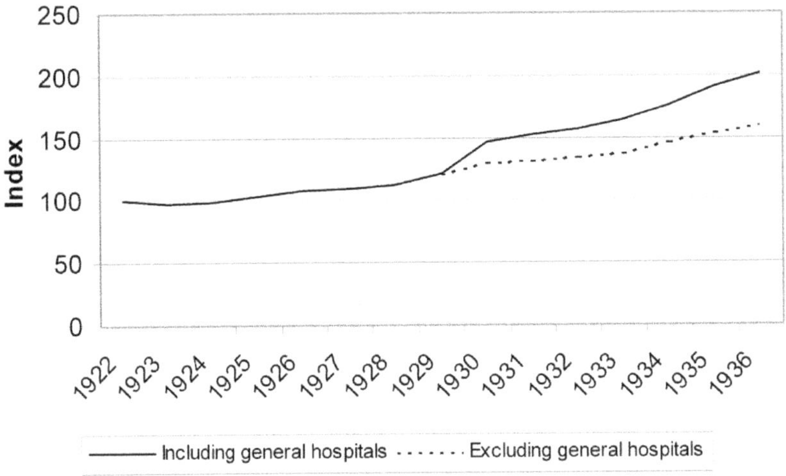

Figure 2.2 Index of County Borough Spending on Public Health Services, 1922/3–36/7
Source: Local Government Financial Statistics, 1922/3–36/7.

Geographical Variations

The data presented so far give clear evidence of an upward trend in investment in municipal health services. As we saw in Chapter One, however, one of the main criticisms of health care before the NHS was its unequal distribution, with some commentators pointing to a north/south divide in particular. This can be examined by breaking down the financial expenditure data further, and taking a regional and then an individual authority approach. Although we will go on to argue that regions are not particularly helpful divisions if we are looking for common experiences, they were units which were commonly used in contemporary investigations. Table 2.1 thus presents some descriptive characteristics of the County Borough expenditure for the period based on the regions recommended by the 1937 Sankey Report on voluntary hospitals. These are also similar to those used by the Ministry of Health and Nuffield Provincial Hospitals Trust when conducting a survey into hospital provision in 1945–6.[9] Expenditure on general hospitals is excluded for the reasons illustrated above. The table shows that there was diversity in the level of expenditure both *between* and *within* regions. When boroughs are ranked by their average level of expenditure over the period, Yorkshire and the East Midlands emerge as the 'best' regions (they have the highest mean ranking of their constituent boroughs). The North East, the North West and the Home Counties are the worst regions on the same score. However, there was significant variation within each region as shown in the diversity between the highest and lowest ranked position in each case: none were made up of consistently highly or poorly ranked authorities. The greatest variation is seen in the West Midlands and Yorkshire, while the least is in the North East, South West and Home Counties.

9 Frazer, *A History of English Public Health*, 450; Ministry of Health, Nuffield Provincial Hospital Trust Hospital Survey (London, 1945–6). As Table 2.1 indicates, there was great variation in the number of County Boroughs in each region.

	East	East Midlands (inc Sheffield)	Home Counties	South-East	North East	North West	South West	West Midlands	Yorkshire	Wales
Mean ranking	37	26.6	52.5	35.5	55.1	46	39.2	60.4	21.9	38.3
Standard Deviation	31.1	16.5	12.0	27.1	18.9	24.4	15.4	59	35	14.9
Coefficient of variation (%)	84.1	62.0	22.9	76.3	34.3	53.0	39.3	114.2	166.7	
Highest ranked borough	Ipswich (10)	Rotherham (4)	Reading (44)	West Ham (2)	Newcastle (23)	Liverpool (1)	Plymouth (27)	Birmingham (14)	Leeds (5)	Swansea (15)
Lowest ranked borough	Gt Yarmouth (71)	Derby (53)	Oxford (61)	Portsmouth (82)	West Hartlepool (78)	Bolton (81)	Bath (66)	Dudley (83)	Dewsbury (40)	Merthyr (79)
N Boroughs	3	9	2	11	8	22	5	11	8	4

Table 2.1 Geographic Breakdown of Average County Borough Expenditure on Health, 1922/3–36/7 (excluding general hospitals)
Source: Local Government Financial Statistics, 1922/3–36/7.

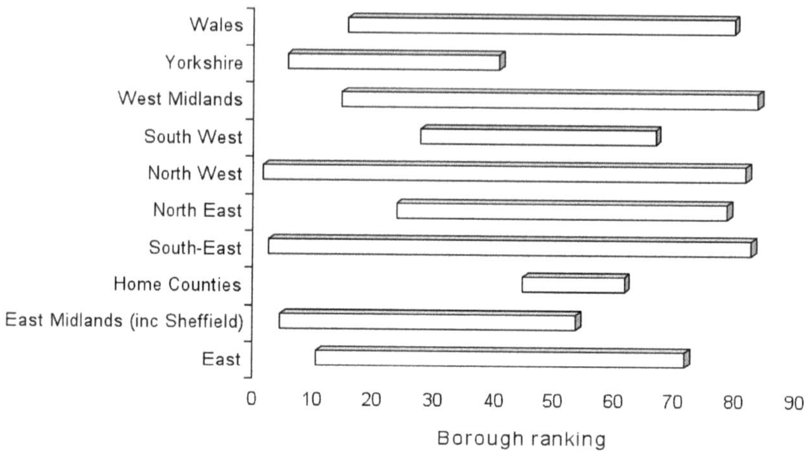

Figure 2.3 Spread of Rankings on Health Expenditure by Region, 1922/3–36/7 (excluding general hospitals)

Source: Local Government Financial Statistics, 1922/3–36/7.

It is difficult to see a clear picture as the crude statistics sometimes point in different directions, but it is evident that a straightforward north-south divide is too simplistic. In particular, some 'northern' regions such as the North West and Yorkshire were broadly high spenders, while the (admittedly small) Home Counties region is a low spender. There was also significant variation within regions as suggested by two measures of dispersion. The difference between the highest and lowest ranked boroughs (illustrated in Figure 2.3) simply gives information on the two extreme observations, while the coefficient of variation and the standard deviation (the degree of spread – both indicated in Table 2.1) is based on all observations. Descriptive statistics for the low numbers in this dataset must be treated with some caution, but it can be seen from Figure 2.3 that the North East tended to feature towards the bottom part of the distribution, while the North West and the South East covered almost the entire range. The Yorkshire county boroughs, meanwhile, clustered in the top part of the range.

The two measures of dispersal based on the data variation within each region (the coefficient of variation and the standard deviation) add to this picture. The North East showed a low degree of dispersal, for example, while Yorkshire and the West Midlands had high levels of variation. For many regions, however, one or two leading centres raised the average ranking for the region as a whole. For example, the North-West contained Liverpool (ranked 1) and Manchester (8), along with the smaller boroughs of Chester (12) and Salford (13), bringing up the mean level of spending. Coexisting with these high spending boroughs, however, were those such as Blackburn (ranked 73), Bury (69), Carlisle (68), Oldham (74), Preston (75) and Bolton (81). In other cases the leading centres were not so highly ranked themselves, and failed to drag up the regional average – given the presence also of many low spending councils in the same region. Regions in this position include the West Midlands, where the largest centre (Birmingham) was ranked 14th, and lay alongside low ranking boroughs like such as Coventry (ranked 80), Smethwick (77) and Wolverhampton (76). The North-East was in a similar situation, top ranking Newcastle (23) coexisting with West Hartlepool (78) and Tynemouth (72).

Several of the remaining areas contained only very few County Boroughs (the Home Counties, the East, the South-West and Wales), and the descriptive characteristics may be misleading as indicators of healthcare provision. The Home County towns of Reading and Oxford to the west of London were low ranked, for example (44 and 61 respectively), but both contained flourishing voluntary organisations, which may have lessened the need to spend highly on municipal health services.[10] Oxford was, however, among the County Boroughs characterised by J. P. Bradbury as having 'simply opted not to provide good all-round services'.[11] The South-Western

10 M. Gorsky, J. Mohan and M. Powell, 'British Voluntary Hospitals, 1871–1938: The Geography of Provision and Utilization', *Journal of Historical Geography*, 25 (1999).

11 J. P. Bradbury, 'The 1929 Local Government Act: The Formulation and Implementation of Poor Law (Health Care) and Exchequer Grants Reform for England and Wales (Outside London)', PhD Thesis, University of Bristol, 1991, 304; E. Peretz, 'The Costs of Modern Motherhood to Low Income Families in Interwar Britain', in V. A. Fildes,

region was in a similar situation, with boroughs such as Bath supporting extensive voluntary associations. The last region is the South-East, which was a large group of boroughs extending to the south coast from the greater London area.[12] This was a region with a particularly large degree of internal diversity. It contained variously high spending boroughs which were really part of the London conurbation, such as West Ham (ranked 2) and Croydon (28), and rich seaside resorts and cathedral towns such as Eastbourne (3) and Canterbury (18), alongside overcrowded, poor boroughs adjoining London such as East Ham (7), and low-spending port and seaside towns like Brighton (63), Portsmouth (82) and Bournemouth (58), all on the south coast. This is reflected in the extreme range of rankings, from 2 to 82, showing virtually all the national variation in one region, and highlighting the lack of regional uniformity in the Ministry's own scheme.

It is clear, therefore, that there was substantial geographic variation across England and Wales in terms of expenditure on health. While there are some suggestions of a north/south divide, the evidence points more strongly to a lack of uniformity of experience within many of the regions used in official enquiries, with some high spending northern boroughs and some low spending southern boroughs.[13] Some examples have suggested that this could be due to well developed voluntary medical sectors. In other cases, however, the overall ranking may have disguised a variety of attitudes to investment in different aspects of municipal health care, a consideration to which we turn in the next section.

L. Marks and H. Marland, eds, *Women and Children First: International Maternal and Infant Welfare, 1870–1945* (London, 1992); E. Peretz, 'Infant Welfare Between the Wars', in R. C. Whiting ed., *Oxford: Studies in the History of a University Town since 1800* (Manchester, 1993).

12 This region is called 'London' in the 1945–6 Ministry of Health, Nuffield Provincial Hospital Trust Survey, but since we are not considering the Metropolitan boroughs, we have re-named it for clarity's sake.

13 M. Powell, 'A Tale of Two Cities: a Critical Evaluation of the Geographic Provision of Health Care Before the NHS', *Public Administration*, 70 (Spring, 1992), also notes that 'while ... the south did tend to have more beds than the north, the North-West region was relatively well provided with 6.7 beds per thousand population, making it second only to the London region for these categories' (73).

Variations Between Sectors

Much of the historical debate has been conducted at the level of total expenditure at one point in time. However, as our analysis has started to suggest, these figures can mask significant variation over time. The same is true of patterns of individual (sub-sector) health services in different boroughs, as we will go on to show. Once again, therefore, taking an aggregate view disguises the prioritisation and decision making which went on in different boroughs.[14]

Even at a national level, trends of expenditure varied considerably from one sub-sector to another. Figure 2.4 illustrates these trends for the major personal health services, averaged across all County Boroughs. Spending on TB and infectious disease schemes were about four times as high, per capita, as those for mental deficiency and VD, for example. Furthermore, some services, like mental hospitals and provision for infectious diseases, attracted fairly flat levels of investment over the period, while others increased enormously. Spending on MCW, for example, doubled to become the second highest funded service and that on mental deficiency increased fivefold to overtake mental hospitals. General hospitals formed another case apart, as has already been noted, driving most of the aggregate spike in expenditure in 1930. In fact, spending on general hospitals accounted for about half of total health spending in 1930.

14 A few other authors have pointed to the influence of local circumstances on expenditure decisions, although they have not taken this to a sub-sectoral level. For examples, see, L. J. Sharpe and K. Newton, *Does Politics Matter? The Determinants of Public Policy* (Oxford, 1984); J. R. Hicks and U. K. Hicks, 'Standards of Local Expenditure: A Problem of the Inequality of Incomes', *Occasional Papers*, National Institute of Economic and Social Research (Cambridge, 1943).

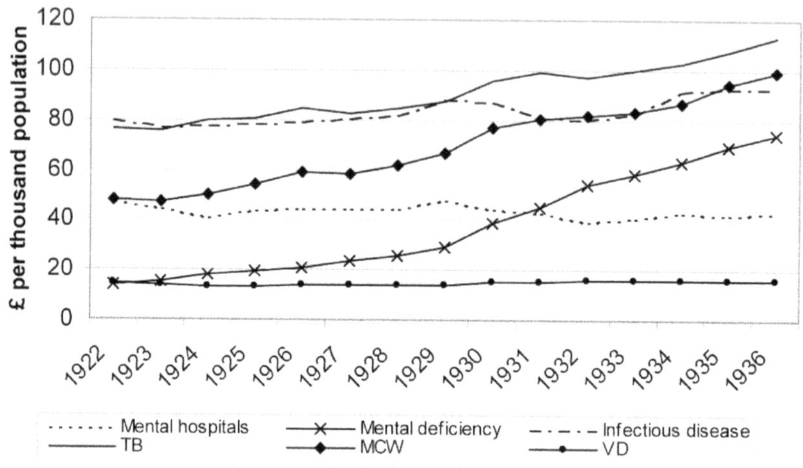

Figure 2.4 Mean County Borough Expenditure per Thousand on Selected Health Services, 1922/3–36/7
Source: Local Government Financial Statistics, 1922/3–36/7.

The aggregated trends by service shown in Figure 2.4 reflect wider commitments in the field of healthcare. The rising levels of expenditure on MCW and mental deficiency, in particular, were at least partly a response to legislative demands such as the 1918 Maternity and Child Welfare Act, the 1913 Mental Deficiency Act, and the 1927 Mental Deficiency Amendment Act. The transfer of mentally defective patients from the Poor Law under the Local Government Act was probably also responsible for raised expenditure under the health remit. Investment in other services such as VD schemes and mental hospitals remained static because they were not current priorities in terms of legislative focus or need.[15] Infectious disease

15 The Minister of Health noted in his Annual Reports of the period that the total number of new cases of VD was falling, although the number of attendances by confirmed sufferers was increasing. In the report for 1931–2, the Minister cited a 46.8 per cent reduction in syphilis cases since 1920 (Ministry of Health Annual Report, 1931–2, 60–1). In 1920, 1,489,000 people attended local authority VD centres (Ministry of Health Annual Report, 1920–1, 11).

hospitals did receive a boost in investment around 1929, like the more rapidly expanding services, but this was not sustained over the remainder of the period, reflecting the move away from epidemic disease to preventive services. The TB services attracted consistently high levels of investment, and rapidly outstripped infectious disease to become the leading sector in terms of expenditure per head until general hospitals came under public health in 1930.

Table 2.2 and Figure 2.5, however, illustrate that these patterns by sector were not all uniform across the dataset. This is shown in the values for the coefficient of variation for each service in Table 2.2, and the size of the error bars in Figure 2.5. Both of these indicators show the dispersal in expenditure from the mean. In particular, where these two figures show increasing dispersal (for example, the size of the error bars gets larger), we can conclude that County Boroughs were showing a greater degree of diversity relative to average spending. We can thus see that expenditure on mental deficiency in particular showed an increasing amount of variation across the boroughs over the period, although the index of spending fell. Some boroughs clearly retained this service as a priority, for whatever reason. The remaining services displayed less diversity over the period, although all showed rising index values, but all have large error bars and coefficients of variation. This may reflect the permissive nature of much of the legislation covering these services.

		1922	1923	1924	1925	1926	1927
Mental hospitals	Mean	47.5	44.6	41.2	43.6	44.5	44.2
	Index	100	94.0	86.8	91.9	93.8	93.1
	CV	88.7	88.7	97.1	95.7	95.0	99.6
Mental deficiency	Mean	13.8	15.4	17.7	19.2	20.6	23.5
	Index	100	111.6	128.7	139.3	149.5	170.6
	CV	77.3	68.9	70.2	72.2	75.6	72.6
Infectious disease	Mean	79.6	76.9	77.8	78.5	79.2	80.2
	Index	100	96.6	97.8	98.5	99.5	100.7
	CV	44.9	54.6	44.1	39.7	44.1	42.5
TB	Mean	76.6	75.9	79.6	80.7	84.4	82.8
	Index	100	99.1	104.0	105.5	110.3	108.2
	CV	53.8	48.3	49.0	46.8	45.7	43.8
MCW	Mean	47.7	47.5	50.1	53.9	58.6	58.2
	Index	100	99.5	105.0	113.0	122.8	121.9
	CV	47.0	46.1	44.6	45.3	44.2	42.0
General hospitals	Mean						
	Index						
	CV						
Total	Mean	334.2	325.1	332.8	346.6	361.8	366.9
	Index	100	97.3	99.6	103.7	108.2	109.8
	CV	30.4	27.3	26.8	25.9	25.4	25.4

1928	1929	1930	1931	1932	1933	1934	1935	1936
44.4	47.7	44.1	42.8	39.9	40.6	43.3	42.5	43.1
93.6	100.5	92.8	90.3	84.0	85.5	91.3	89.6	90.9
106.2	103.7	90.7	87.9	92.8	94.5	90.7	95.8	108.7
25.7	29.1	39.2	44.9	54.1	58.5	63.1	69.6	74.3
186.8	211.8	284.7	326.1	393.0	424.9	458.8	505.8	540.0
67.5	67.1	55.2	55.7	68.2	74.1	71.5	66.7	62.7
81.8	87.9	87.5	81.3	80.1	82.3	91.9	92.6	93.1
102.7	110.4	109.9	102.2	100.7	103.3	115.4	116.3	116.9
43.0	48.4	45.8	45.6	42.6	36.9	36.7	36.4	36.4
84.4	87.5	95.8	98.9	97.4	100.1	102.5	107.8	112.8
110.2	114.3	125.1	129.2	127.2	130.8	133.9	140.8	147.4
44.2	44.0	38.0	33.8	36.9	34.8	35.5	35.5	34.7
61.6	66.5	77.3	80.7	81.8	83.2	86.7	94.7	99.0
129.1	139.3	162.0	169.1	171.4	174.3	181.7	198.4	207.5
40.4	41.6	37.3	39.6	37.7	38.1	37.1	36.7	38.1
		250.9	228.9	222.0	234.4	247.2	286.8	307.5
		100	91.2	88.5	93.4	98.5	114.3	122.6
		58.9	71.1	71.2	63.8	61.4	56.5	51.9
377.9	406.8	488.7	508.3	524.6	549.7	586.3	638.5	671.1
113.1	121.7	146.2	152.1	157.0	164.5	175.4	191.0	200.8
24.8	25.2	30.9	32.7	33.1	31.6	32.3	34.4	34.5

Table 2.2 Mean Expenditure per Thousand on Major Health Services, 1922/3–36/7: Descriptive Statistics

Source: Local Government Financial Statistics, 1922/3–36/7. CV: Coefficient of variation

a) Mental Hospitals

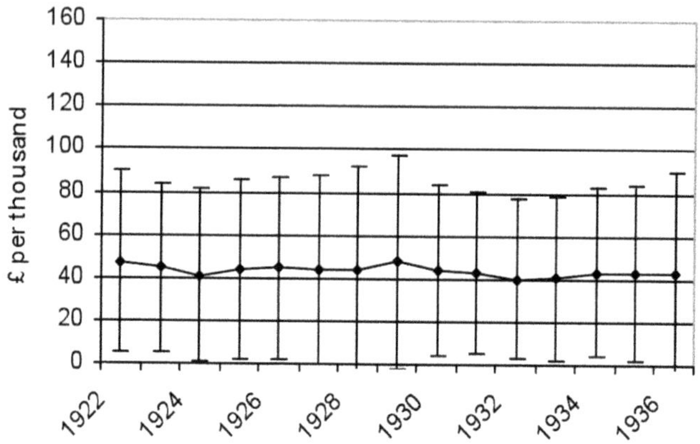

b) Mental Deficiency

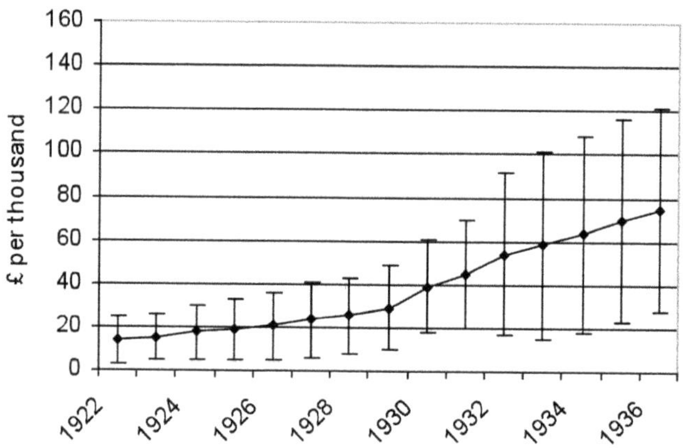

c) Infectious Disease

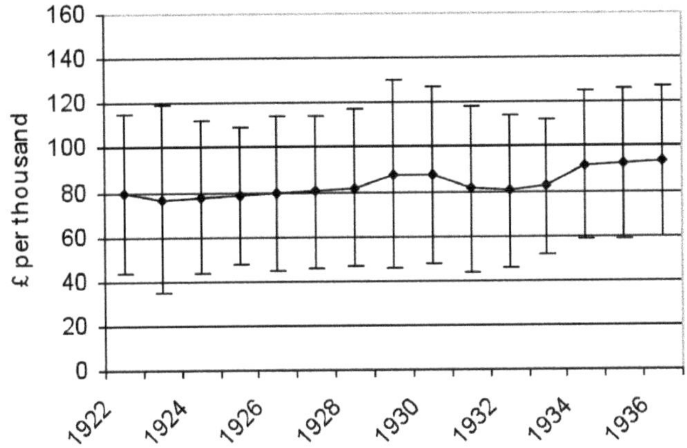

d) TB

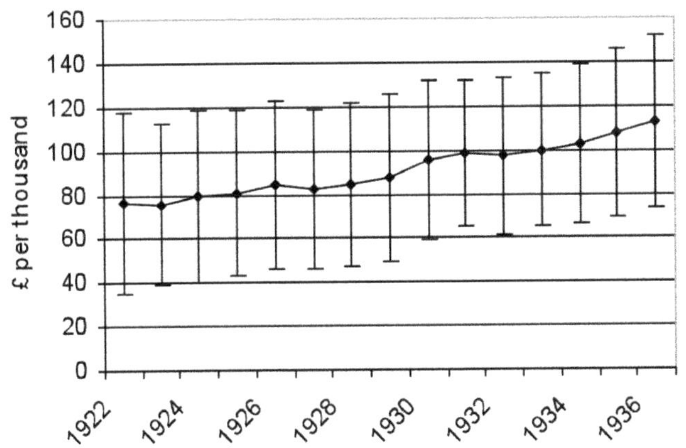

e) MCW

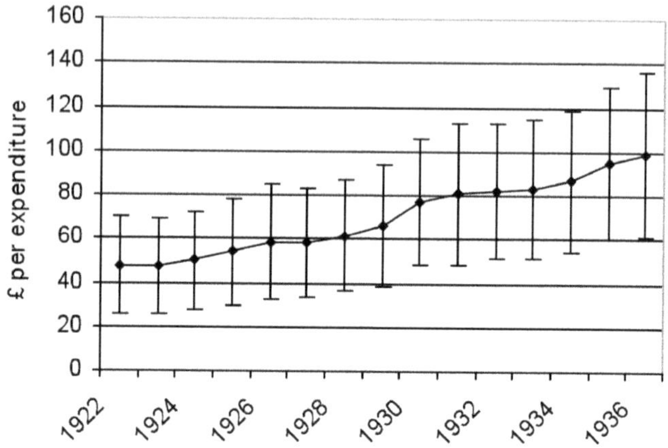

Figure 2.5 Mean County Borough Expenditure per Thousand on Major Health Services, 1922/3–36/7
Source: Local Government Financial Statistics, 1922/3–36/7

This variety in spending by sector can be explored in greater detail by using correlation analysis. This addresses whether boroughs prioritised some services over others: rather than considering each borough's performance relative to the average, we now measure its own investment in each service compared to the other services. To do this, we have calculated correlation coefficients for annual expenditure on different services on a year-by-year basis. This quantifies how far common patterns between sectors existed. A high coefficient would indicate that there was a strong common relationship between the boroughs' expenditure levels on different services in a particular year. The calculation of these coefficients over the interwar period produced a total of over 650 correlations (thirty-six correlations per year prior to 1930 and fifty-five per year subsequently). A summary is offered in Table 2.3, which sets out the number of coefficients which were significant at a 95 per cent level or higher (that is, we can be at least 95 per cent confident that the relationship did not occur by chance).

While there are discernible relationships between services, the coefficients are relatively low, although frequently statistically significant. This supports the considerable degree of variation within the dataset which has already been illustrated, and that high (or low) expenditure on one service did not always correspond with high (or low) expenditure on another, although the tendency is in this direction. Table 2.3 also indicates that the health service appearing most frequently in the list of highest correlations was TB, and its most consistently significant positive relationships were with MCW and disease notification. The strength of the association with MCW increased after 1930, reaching its high of 0.41 in 1932. This is another indication that TB and MCW services were both growing priorities of health care in this period, and both received growing levels of investment across County Boroughs. Given that they were covered by separate pieces of legislation, we may assume that their common trends were the result of elective affinities rather than directed by legislative requirements. Central government certainly held both services as priorities in the interwar period, making it clear that all boroughs were expected to provide access to care for mothers and infants, and for tuberculous patients. The common presence of disease notification may reflect its growing stringency. Expenditure on TB seems to have particularly reflected the aggregate mean trend, given its high level of correlation with several other services. It may also be significant that it was the largest of the individual health services in terms of expenditure, as well as one which particularly mirrored contemporary health concerns.

	Total number of correlations	Proportion of significant correlations (total) (%)*	Proportion of negative correlations (%)*
1922	36	22.2	25.0
1923	36	11.1	27.8
1924	36	19.4	27.8
1925	36	27.8	36.1
1926	36	22.2	36.1
1927	36	22.2	36.1
1928	36	22.2	38.3
1929	36	13.9	38.9
1930	55	16.4	47.3
1931	55	16.4	45.5
1932	55	7.3	43.6
1933	55	12.7	47.3
1934	55	10.9	49.1
1935	55	7.3	32.7
1936	55	7.3	34.5

Proportion of significant negative correlations (%)*	Most significant positive correlation	Most significant negative correlation
0	0.420 (TB x ID)	-0.123 (Misc and Mental hospitals)
0	0.330 (VD x Misc)	-0.121 (Misc and Mental hospitals)
0	0.353 (TB x Mental deficiency)	-0.126 (Notification and Mental hospitals)
0	0.315 (TB x ID)	-0.157 (Misc and Mental hospitals)
0	0.338 (TB x Notification)	-0.174 (Misc and Mental hospitals)
0	0.384 (TB x Notification)	-0.133 (Misc and Mental hospitals)
0	0.380 (TB x Notification)	-0.188 (Misc and Mental hospitals)
0	0.370 (TB x Notification)	-0.193 (Misc and Mental hospitals)
1.8	0.359 (TB x ID)	-0.254 (Salaries and Mental hospitals)
3.6	0.391 (TB x Infectious disease)	-0.229 (Salaries and Mental hospitals)
1.8	0.412 (TB x MCW)	-0.262 (Salaries and Notification)
3.6	0.321 (TB x MCW)	-0.285 (Salaries and Notification)
3.6	0.370 (TB x MCW)	-0.300 (Salaries and Notification)
1.8	0.386 (ID x MCW)	-0.230 (Salaries and Mental hospitals)
0	0.436 (ID x MCW)	-0.224 (General hospitals and MCW)

Table 2.3 Summary of Expenditure Correlations, 1922/3–36/7
*significant at a 95 per cent level of confidence
Source: Local Government Financial Statistics, 1922/3–36/7.

The relatively low correlation coefficients indicate that although expenditure on MCW, TB, and mental deficiency showed a common pattern of growth in the aggregate, this was not uniform across the County Boroughs. In some cases however, such as the schemes for TB and MCW, and to a lesser extent, TB and VD, the strength of the relationship improved after 1929, suggesting that these services received a common boost, either through the new grant system, or through the impetus towards an improved and more unified general health policy. In other cases, such as the relationship between mental deficiency and other health services, the association became less clear after 1929. Mental hospitals were conspicuous in their lack of positive relationships with other services, the only significant correlations being negative ones with salaries from 1930 onwards. Mental hospitals appeared in only five significant correlations (all negative), compared with forty-nine for TB (forty-eight of them positive), and thirty-seven for infectious disease (all positive). This confirms that there was not large-scale investment in mental hospitals at this time, in contrast with other parts of the municipal health service.[16] The changes in the strength of relationships between spending on different services therefore indicates changing health priorities, as some services such as infectious disease hospitals waned, while others such as MCW reached maturity. It is worth noting that while, as indicated in Table 2.3, there were often a considerable number of negative

16 Elsewhere, we note that mental hospitals did attract a high level of capital investment in this period, despite the generally low expenditure from the revenue accounts (A. Levene, M. Powell and J. Stewart, 'Patterns of Municipal Health Expenditure in Interwar England and Wales', *Bulletin of the History of Medicine*, 78 (2004), 650. The mental health services had their roots much further back in time than many of the services which were expanding in the interwar period, and this may have impeded their development in the 1920s and 1930s. Philo notes the widespread network of mental asylums which were set up in Britain in the nineteenth century, in a deliberate attempt to minimise the amount of 'distance-decay' in their usage. C. Philo, 'Journey to Asylum: A Medical-Geographical Idea in Historical Context', *Journal of Historical Geography*, 21:2 (1995). This network, which placed asylums in local centres of population may have meant that they fell under the responsibility of the administrative county rather than being in the centre of towns and therefore falling to the County Boroughs. This may partly account for the uneven pattern of development of mental hospitals in the interwar period.

relationships between services, they were rarely significant. Apart from the coefficients concerning mental hospitals and general hospitals, commented on above and below, most involved minor services such as miscellaneous health, and salaries. Almost all of the few significant negative relationships were between salaries and mental hospitals, rather than between any of the major services. The overall trend was, therefore, towards common expenditure patterns within boroughs on a year by year basis.

Although the newly transferred service of general hospitals was well correlated in trend over time with the other services, relationships with other services across the boroughs which appropriated an institution from the Public Assistance into the Public Health remit on a year-by-year basis were weak. Coefficients were often negative, although they did not reach the 95 per cent significance level. This suggests that, generally, boroughs which spent highly on general hospitals tended to spend less on services such as VD and TB, perhaps because they integrated these into the general hospital structure, or because the total money available was limited. The state of the buildings inherited from the Poor Law was a significant factor in the level of required investment, as well as the ability and inclination of the borough to invest. It is thus not very surprising that this service followed a different course from some of the others, but it illustrates again the need to disaggregate general hospitals from the more general picture of municipal health care. The development of general hospitals as part of boroughs' wider health policy will be considered in Chapter Three.

The correlation data therefore suggest that investment in some health services began to follow a common course in the second half of the period, while others experienced the opposite effect. Table 2.3 showed that the proportion of significant correlations fell, but this is partly because the pool was diluted by two services (general hospitals and also vaccination), which did not follow a similar path to the longer-established sectors. Nevertheless, the high coefficients of variation and large error bars shown in Table 2.2 and Figure 2.5 point to a significant degree of difference between boroughs, suggesting that some were spurred on to respond specifically to local needs by the 1929 Local Government Act. Central priorities may therefore have encouraged broad trends towards expenditure on certain services, which the priorities and circumstances of individual boroughs then mediated into the wide range of expenditure illustrated in our figures.

There was certainly communality of purpose between the designs of central government and local authorities in health care provision, and we should not overstate the degree of grassroots determinism. Nevertheless, the evidence points to a great variety of experience in the levels of investment made in different services. This will be picked up in the case studies in Chapters Four to Seven.

Sub-Sectoral Trends Across the Interwar Period

The evidence considered so far has thus suggested that boroughs did not act uniformly in allocating resources between services although there were certain common trends. In Table 2.5 (at the end of the chapter), we couple the dimension of sub-sectoral variation with a measure of change over time. The left-hand side of the table shows expenditure per thousand population on the five largest health services for each borough in 1936. These data enable us to judge the extent to which boroughs tended to prioritise one or more services, or whether they might be exceptional investors in one, and exceptional under-investors in another. The right-hand side shows the percentage change in the major services from 1922, indicating whether boroughs maintained similar patterns of investment over time. General hospitals are omitted from the right-hand side, since they were not present in the health budget in 1922.

By analysing the data in this way we are able to address the typology of spending. One such influential scheme was set out by the analysts of local government J. R. and U. K. Hicks, writing in the 1940s.[17] They classified boroughs as being either 'spenders' or 'stinters', according to their patterns of investment. An examination of Table 2.5, however, illustrates that a typology which focuses solely on total expenditure at one fixed date is insufficient, as it hides significant variation over time and between sectors. At first glance our data reveal a varied list of high total spenders:

17 Hicks and Hicks, 'Standards of Local Expenditure', 9.

Birmingham, East Ham, Kingston upon Hull, Lincoln, Liverpool, Manchester, Norwich, Rotherham, Swansea, Walsall, West Ham and York. The low spenders or 'stinters' include a similarly diverse list of Blackburn, Bolton, Dudley, Portsmouth, South Shields and Stockport.

Our data allow us to nuance Hicks and Hicks's picture by examining whether boroughs changed over time from being spenders to being stinters or vice versa. We should beware of assuming that the figures represent a continuous trend from 1922 to 1936, but as a crude indicator, they suffice. The mean figures for percentage change since 1922 show a tendency towards increase in all the major services except mental hospitals. Again, however, there is evidence of divergence from the national trend in individual boroughs. In each case, there are examples of boroughs which bucked the trend, and those which display it at an exaggerated level. While the trend in investment on mental hospitals was downward, for example, a number of boroughs – including Smethwick, Burton, Norwich, and Stoke upon Trent – showed significant expansion. Bradford, Bristol, Liverpool, and Grimsby are examples of boroughs showing a percentage decline in spending on infectious disease while the national trend was roughly steady, and Wakefield, Croydon, Liverpool, and Bury (among others) showed a fall off in spending on TB services. No boroughs had a decline in spending between 1922 and 1936 on MCW or mental deficiency. Some, however, expanded more rapidly than others. Worcester, Bradford, Southport, Wallasey, and South Shields, for example, showed a slow expansion in MCW investment, while Halifax, Oldham, Grimsby, Great Yarmouth, and Smethwick forged ahead.

We may also identify boroughs which had a general tendency towards decline in expenditure over the period, and others which were consistent in their expansion. Bradford, Liverpool, Exeter, Eastbourne, Croydon, Canterbury, and Bury all had a tendency to spend less on both TB and infectious disease services; the only services in which decline was evident in this group. Most of these boroughs are notable for being relatively wealthy, and it is possible that their decline relative to 1922 indicates that they started from a high level, and did not need to increase investment to the extent that poorer boroughs might. This is reinforced when the rapidly expanding boroughs are considered: Merthyr Tydfil, Southampton, Swansea, and Walsall; all poorer boroughs which were investing at a low level at the start of the period.

A number of boroughs changed their spending levels over time in a different way from the national trend. This can be seen by examining the z-score (not shown), which denotes a standardized measure of spending relative to the average: a z score of +1.0 suggests spending a standard deviation above the mean, while a score of -1.0 suggests spending a standard deviation below the mean.[18] If we take expenditure on mental hospitals, for example, Canterbury moved from a z-score of 4.6 in 1922 (that is, over four and a half standardized units above the mean) to just above the borough average in 1936. South Shields and West Hartlepool reduced their spending on the same service from above 1.0 to close to -1.0. On the other hand, East Ham increased its expenditure from 2.7 to 6.3 standard units. For mental deficiency, some boroughs increased by over one unit (Bristol, South Shields, Swansea, Walsall, and West Bromwich), while others reduced their spending by the same amount (Bradford, Croydon, Ipswich, Kingston upon Hull, Leeds, Leicester, Oxford, Reading, and York). Similar increases for infectious disease are found for Barnsley, Bath, Burton, Lincoln, Southport, Swansea, Wakefield, Walsall and West Hartlepool, while reductions are seen for Bradford, Bristol, Canterbury, and Liverpool. There are equivalent examples for the other services as well.

However, very few boroughs were high or low spenders on all services. A handful, largely in the economically depressed North-West, did spend below the average on all services for 1936: Blackburn, Blackpool, Bolton, Bury, Carlisle, Dudley, Preston, Stockport, Stoke, Wigan, and Worcester. These boroughs were generally small, and tended to be poor. It is possible that they could not afford to spend at a very high level compared with larger and wealthier boroughs. A smaller number were consistently high spenders in 1936: Cardiff, Norwich, and West Ham. The latter was exceptional in this regard. Leeds and Lincoln only spent below the average on one service (mental hospitals in both cases, which were shown above to have followed a different path of investment from other services). There are many other instances, however, where boroughs were not so clear-cut in their commitment (or otherwise) to health policy in general. Instead,

18 The z-score is derived from the distance of the standard deviation from the mean and is calculated by (n-mean)/standard deviation.

they showed a notable preference for one or more services. Barnsley, for example, was a slightly below average investor in both mental hospitals and mental deficiency, but spent considerably above the mean on infectious disease and MCW. Bath was more polarised, investing notably in infectious disease hospitals, but equally notable in its underinvestment on TB services. Again, other examples make the same point for a variety of different sector combinations.

While regional patterns are not fully clear at the level of total expenditure (see above), it is possible to detect a degree of regional concentration in certain services. Yorkshire, for example, had a slight tendency to spend at above average levels on MCW over the whole period (four out of the fourteen boroughs with very high levels of investment on this service were in Yorkshire). The Southern and South-Eastern boroughs were, with the sole exception of Portsmouth, above-average spenders on mental hospitals. Canterbury, East Ham, Eastbourne, Southampton, and Southend were all notably above-average investors, and the remaining five boroughs were all above the mean. This regional concentration is significant given the lack of notable correlation between mental hospitals and other services at an aggregate level; suggesting more method behind the provision for madness than has hitherto been found. The boroughs in this region were also generally under-investors in MCW services compared to the mean. Five boroughs in the North-West region were notably above the mean in average spending on infectious disease over the period, the general tendency towards stagnation in this service notwithstanding.[19] This may be related to the fact that many of the North-Western boroughs are located on the coast, which might raise their need to prioritise minimising exposure to infectious disease brought in from outside. Not all the high spenders were coastal boroughs, however, and so this may also be a hangover from an earlier focus on epidemic disease as the major scourge to health. The way that the inclinations of individual officers or committees could skew investment will be illustrated particularly forcefully in the case study of Eastbourne County Borough (see Chapter Five).

19 That is, displaying a mean z-score above 1.

A final indication of the need to refine a simple dichotomy of 'spenders' and 'stinters' such as that used by Hicks and Hicks is provided in Table 2.4. Here, we list the top and bottom ten spenders on each service in 1936. Again, we see that few boroughs were consistent spenders or stinters on all services. West Ham, the exceptional spender when compared to the mean, was in the top ten for four services: mental hospitals, TB, mental deficiency, and infectious disease. Liverpool was in the top ten for three services, although one was general hospitals for which there were fewer boroughs making expenditure (the remaining two were TB and MCW). On the other hand, Merthyr Tydfil and Oxford both appear several times in the lowest spender lists: Merthyr for mental hospitals and mental deficiency, and Oxford for mental hospitals, MCW and infectious disease. It is somewhat surprising to see these two boroughs juxtaposed, given their extremely different economic backgrounds. Merthyr was a deprived borough, heavily dependent on coal mining, while Oxford was affluent, with an economy benefiting from new industries such as motorcar manufacture. In Merthyr we may see a lack of interest in mental health services generally, whereas in Oxford (where we have already noted the presence of a lively voluntary sector), deficient spending was carried across services catering for different types of patients. Other boroughs showed a more mixed pattern, and were at the top of the rankings in one sector, but at the bottom on another. West Bromwich, for example, was among the top ten spenders on both mental health services, but in the bottom ten on TB and MCW. The fact that a relatively poorly off borough spent so highly on some services, perhaps to the detriment of others, clearly suggests prioritisation of some sort, and certainly a need to move beyond the simple scheme of authorities inclined to spend or stint.

Highest spenders	*Lowest spenders*	*Highest spenders*	*Lowest spenders*	*Highest spenders*	*Lowest spenders*
Mental hospitals		Mental deficiency		Infectious disease	
East Ham	Dudley	West Bromwich	Great Yarmouth	Barnsley	South Shields
Swansea	Worcester	Walsall	Stockport	Wakefield	Gateshead
Southend	South Shields	Bristol	Stoke	West Ham	Bolton
West Ham	Ipswich	Birmingham	Blackpool	Warrington	Nottingham
Southampton	Merthyr Tydfil	Ipswich	Southport	Southport	Wolverhampton
Northampton	West Hartlepool	Leicester	Warrington	Chester	Oxford
Bournemouth	Blackpool	West Ham	Merthyr Tydfil	Gloucester	Tynemouth
Hastings	Southport	Oxford	Gloucester	Bath	Burnley
Eastbourne	Warrington	Nottingham	Burton	Burton	Northampton
Hull	Oxford	Newcastle	Newport	Doncaster	Dudley
TB		MCW		General Hospitals	
Rotherham	Wakefield	Lincoln	Great Yarmouth	Salford	Hull
Ipswich	Bolton	Wakefield	Southend	Manchester	Swansea
Grimsby	Bath	Hull	Hastings	Rochdale	Southport
Liverpool	Darlington	St Helen's	Oxford	Southend	Bristol
Plymouth	Southend	Liverpool	Brighton	West Bromwich	Coventry
West Ham	West Hartlepool	Swansea	Nottingham	Warrington	Sunderland
Warrington	Portsmouth	Dewsbury	Canterbury	Birkenhead	Middlesborough
East Ham	West Bromwich	Grimsby	Tynemouth	Liverpool	Sheffield
Manchester	Blackpool	Barnsley	South Shields	Halifax	Smethwick
Norwich	Wallasey	Rotherham	West Bromwich	Cardiff	Gloucester

Table 2.4 Highest and Lowest Spenders on Major Health Services, 1936
Source: Local Government Financial Statistics, 1936

Conclusions

The consideration of disaggregated patterns of expenditure by time, geographical location and sector has allowed for a much more nuanced view of local health priorities than that gained from the national, aggregate picture. Correlation analysis has shown that there were common trends in expenditure levels on several services in different boroughs, but that there was a significant amount of variation within the dataset, both when considered at a static point in time, and across the period. This was highlighted in the relatively weak, although statistically significant correlation coefficients, and in both the large error bars seen in Figures 2.1 and 2.5, and the large coefficients of variation in Tables 2.1 and 2.2. The mental health services showed less clear relationships with other services, as did general hospitals. Although the 1929 Local Government Act almost certainly gave an incentive for individual boroughs to invest, and in general terms prompted higher levels of interest in and commitment to municipal health services, there was considerable variation in the way and extent to which this manifested itself at local level. Other, sector-specific legislation may have promoted greater diversity within the dataset because of its generally permissive character, even if a minimum requirement was compulsory. Expenditure on some of these services was also encouraged up to 1929 by large percentage grants.[20] This may account for the different rates of change in different boroughs.

In the aggregate, there was an expansion in expenditure on most services over time, with some tendency towards convergence of experience across the County Boroughs. The analysis of individual cases, however, allows us to highlight a considerable degree of difference in behaviour across the interwar period. There are examples of boroughs which were consistently high or low spenders on all fronts, such as West Ham and Wigan respectively. We have also demonstrated, however, that we need a more nuanced view of spending patterns than the simple dichotomy set up by Hicks and Hicks between

20 Expenditure on MCW services was matched by a 50 per cent grant from 1915, and that on mental deficiency from 1916. VD schemes attracted a 75 per cent grant from 1916. In 1921, a 50 per cent grant was attached to expenditure on TB services. M. Newcomer, *Central and Local Finance in Germany and England* (New York, 1937), 346–7.

'spenders' and 'stinters'. Instead, many boroughs invested particularly heavily or deficiently in one or more services over time, indicating that some discretion was left to individual councils or officers. This highlights that a borough's reputation as a spender or stinter may be very much affected by the use of total rather than sub-sectoral expenditure data, and also the period under study. A static picture will not necessarily provide a true representation of investment over time. Bradford, for example, was a high spender at the start of the period, but moved closer to the mean over the course of the interwar period. Swansea and Merthyr moved in the opposite direction.

It is unwise to place too much emphasis on local choices and preferences, however. Complete local determinism was impossible, given the need and obligation to provide what the Ministry judged to be a sufficient level of care in different areas. This may have been especially true in the 1930s, when the Ministry was using its surveys of local standards of health services to prompt investment in particular areas.[21] Even prior to this, however, the annual central audit of local financial returns may have flagged up boroughs which were especially niggardly or lavish. Having said all that, it is evident that prioritisation did take place, albeit within certain bounds. An enthusiastic public health officer might do much for investment in his own area of interest, as occurred in the well documented case of Rochdale with regard to MCW services in the 1930s.[22] Other council members might also affect levels of expenditure on particular services, especially if they had an influence over the setting of the budget. In short, our analysis of expenditure on the interwar health services has revealed the variety of experiences in the national dataset, showing different patterns of growth and decline over time, over space and between sectors. It is clear that studying expenditure at the aggregate level reveals only a crude, static and dichotomous picture, which fails to capture the complex and nuanced picture of provision. In the next chapter we will start to unpick the underlying reasons behind these varied stories of investment and neglect.

21 See Chapters One and Three.

22 An intensive campaign in Rochdale in the 1930s to increase obstetric care resulted in a much lowered rate of maternal mortality. I. Loudon, 'Some International Features of Maternal Mortality, 1880–1950', in V. A. Fildes, L. Marks and H. Marland, eds, *Women and Children First*, 15.

	Expenditure per thousand in 1936						Change from 1922				
	Mental hospitals	Mental deficiency	Infectious disease	TB	MCW	Total expenditure minus general hospitals	Mental hospitals	Mental deficiency	Infectious disease	TB	MCW
Barnsley	20.55	50.28	212.05	113.22	144.62	647.76	34.10	75.46	40.45	37.36	49.55
Barrow	19.79	49.64	93.63	97.84	125.29	516.39	-107.13	83.95	34.26	14.53	55.88
Bath	49.54	74.81	139.04	51.90	116.60	506.29	28.77	65.20	69.85	29.14	54.43
Birkenhead	28.45	68.18	74.80	80.84	65.14	445.45	-37.88	77.80	23.79	17.70	43.74
Birmingham	49.28	165.41	109.05	107.22	139.73	691.11	6.28	84.15	36.01	13.85	64.33
Blackburn	23.84	53.97	60.56	91.78	80.54	406.40	-101.42	82.63	-14.58	34.23	52.99
Blackpool	12.74	31.27	77.44	75.56	91.64	459.12	-203.57	76.51	-23.14	13.77	32.57
Bolton	22.63	56.74	43.64	46.82	68.59	348.00	-142.67	81.15	14.74	14.22	50.86
Bootle	19.92	48.32	93.57	114.04	106.72	497.42	-146.84	82.33	30.82	18.82	60.32
Bournemouth	77.46	59.26	127.07	77.50	88.83	530.03	22.89	87.56	34.51	24.14	74.49
Bradford	31.02	88.65	88.91	114.13	124.15	574.73	3.36	63.43	-157.24	-10.42	10.88
Brighton	66.34	69.61	63.36	94.90	48.68	411.46	-15.87	85.74	-32.26	5.73	53.74
Bristol	21.01	174.75	61.01	133.15	88.61	569.01	50.98	86.44	-74.27	29.47	63.24
Burnley	21.64	54.27	53.82	111.26	130.61	497.06	-120.73	82.77	3.29	42.99	34.11
Burton	19.59	37.51	137.85	114.22	83.72	544.59	98.66	60.89	48.84	55.02	50.49
Bury	16.35	41.03	60.67	77.08	68.89	426.68	-93.34	85.05	-33.52	-30.37	49.68
Canterbury	49.29	77.50	94.17	94.40	50.48	459.48	-391.57	80.06	-26.02	-11.61	51.39

Table 2.5 Expenditure per Thousand on Major Health Services, 1936/7, and Percentage Change From 1922/3
Source: Local Government Financial Statistics, 1922/3 and 1936/7

Cardiff	51.00	77.92	115.30	149.32	116.18	610.11	-177.77	80.57	43.29	79.97	60.66
Carlisle	15.48	70.61	56.67	92.16	90.61	448.52	4.37	94.76	38.47	21.25	41.84
Chester	63.61	102.19	145.49	131.35	79.08	636.79	25.47	86.27	27.64	32.37	65.37
Coventry	31.22	39.05	96.26	99.10	65.90	423.96	40.38	82.06	18.72	76.63	24.43
Croydon	40.69	61.54	91.58	94.36	87.19	455.12	-88.33	54.87	-23.51	-32.52	50.68
Darlington	22.25	69.10	127.07	54.01	88.08	439.14	18.82	94.86	25.45	8.39	29.81
Derby	48.94	49.15	108.89	144.86	123.83	585.24	60.35	64.06	26.38	55.37	73.85
Dewsbury	20.70	66.45	113.04	103.01	153.99	561.02	-12.07	81.18	5.63	44.55	74.03
Doncaster*	18.49	52.68	137.23	102.07	100.54	519.29	-51.77	47.88	46.75	45.45	22.11
Dudley	0.00	60.16	55.09	82.42	77.22	382.36	**	80.18	87.36	81.74	50.81
East Ham	341.21	96.48	132.68	166.67	77.69	916.85	52.07	81.28	13.21	39.85	49.66
Eastbourne	76.01	57.87	90.56	94.53	122.11	493.11	-164.99	73.48	-10.15	-16.98	20.50
Exeter	22.94	82.21	83.57	103.96	81.24	464.17	7.64	82.62	-4.25	-4.08	68.97
Gateshead	44.02	57.92	42.87	130.58	81.25	500.41	-12.90	98.66	37.53	43.81	50.74
Gloucester	37.73	36.21	142.85	105.99	74.10	473.26	49.29	68.27	5.91	64.51	34.12
Grimsby	27.93	55.80	60.68	212.67	152.33	607.20	18.04	99.47	-34.86	74.17	76.92
Gt Yarmouth	69.78	21.70	98.48	126.71	31.88	449.53	60.95	96.51	-5.26	48.03	76.10
Halifax	36.27	70.88	133.07	97.83	123.26	604.49	8.20	71.08	31.01	26.49	84.99
Hastings	76.24	78.52	91.29	89.66	46.32	478.16	-3.69	78.66	19.24	4.28	55.15
Huddersfield	26.41	40.66	103.04	108.30	105.69	478.41	-2.77	68.97	-13.61	30.59	72.29
Ipswich	6.00	128.23	99.81	218.11	92.69	626.73	100.00	69.21	1.25	10.56	55.35
Kingston upon Hull	75.77	64.32	105.17	98.09	175.43	678.53	59.44	49.50	47.39	37.25	69.51

* Doncaster became a county borough in 1927. Percentage change figures are calculated from 1927.

** Dudley did not spend on mental hospitals from 1931 onwards.

Leeds	34.06	96.33	110.56	151.22	112.46	649.07		-21.67	59.16	-27.41	33.72	30.33
Leicester	30.28	123.43	72.01	129.70	84.03	564.38		3.08	61.63	39.37	46.71	19.37
Lincoln	38.88	81.87	117.25	149.62	228.11	750.09		40.06	97.01	55.37	21.98	50.87
Liverpool	34.22	66.36	122.94	208.36	166.57	729.07		-127.97	81.40	-41.62	-30.98	35.49
Manchester	23.12	57.99	93.22	166.36	122.53	658.75		-126.81	84.32	-12.87	33.88	40.96
Merthyr Tydfil	7.56	35.66	135.53	94.18	112.61	438.48		-65.82	91.45	23.09	85.14	57.68
Middlesbrough	22.77	62.34	134.04	100.53	93.96	576.50		-95.79	88.81	28.02	63.63	32.80
Newcastle	19.12	111.40	112.35	120.70	94.96	552.19		-272.04	79.84	17.32	20.03	61.21
Newport	51.06	38.16	98.07	131.78	107.90	524.69		-39.95	85.86	19.76	82.56	62.93
Northampton	92.07	40.56	55.08	106.60	67.23	441.28		21.73	88.33	-2.16	24.86	54.84
Norwich	57.63	95.13	107.03	161.66	137.36	681.34		78.30	76.91	7.61	65.80	71.69
Nottingham	58.48	115.77	44.34	103.17	49.06	605.87		56.75	87.02	28.33	54.34	36.07
Oldham	18.65	46.77	82.07	91.70	130.18	479.07		-66.94	87.07	18.28	37.75	84.66
Oxford	14.50	120.38	45.23	78.23	46.54	430.00		-310.43	54.89	-27.35	61.09	71.41
Plymouth	28.40	83.16	72.93	196.76	70.57	540.01		-1.40	80.41	14.37	51.02	63.04
Portsmouth	33.77	75.86	77.15	65.62	69.67	400.00		11.67	83.37	2.67	45.36	59.09
Preston	18.17	42.27	62.80	99.96	80.85	415.95		-175.25	77.77	13.24	44.93	61.68
Reading	33.13	61.78	74.89	101.75	128.71	474.19		-13.06	46.21	0.20	35.49	30.95
Rochdale	15.60	39.13	86.06	120.70	121.14	485.77		-72.57	86.66	-4.39	1.43	36.56
Rotherham	23.20	59.25	80.61	222.62	141.21	652.31		-22.15	90.36	2.11	29.00	56.81
Salford	32.25	67.45	120.78	125.37	82.31	589.51		-87.10	83.42	-12.34	32.56	37.77
Sheffield	33.17	80.30	93.81	159.18	110.35	590.52		4.88	73.82	9.48	30.65	60.56

Note: Mean and standard deviation figures have not been calculated for total expenditure minus general hospitals in 1936 because the latter category was not a uniform head of expenditure across the whole dataset.

Smethwick	37.63	80.52	65.39	86.79	116.83	461.52		99.49	84.90	-4.12	15.51	74.52
South Shields	1.94	74.52	41.39	119.54	61.05	381.52		-5107.64	96.11	-30.78	40.20	17.97
Southampton	107.62	105.68	82.04	143.04	90.98	605.10		23.47	97.57	10.20	58.05	65.18
Southend	176.06	42.78	75.91	54.97	33.01	456.58		16.83	72.57	-0.68	4.27	45.60
Southport	13.65	34.25	147.60	81.62	89.98	480.65		-103.88	84.80	57.38	-8.45	13.50
St Helens	17.46	43.12	95.94	127.11	172.49	581.31		-47.68	88.47	36.49	26.42	47.53
Stockport	17.42	27.98	83.87	92.42	88.59	382.82		-142.18	93.01	26.64	31.22	66.24
Stoke on Trent	39.97	30.94	81.05	96.01	90.77	433.05		74.42	64.49	-1.03	49.69	51.38
Sunderland	25.54	68.01	62.35	138.51	86.11	466.57		-21.50	91.95	-1.62	59.89	46.70
Swansea	193.27	70.92	113.50	122.97	166.47	768.09		44.55	99.56	48.51	79.92	71.33
Tynemouth	14.78	89.58	50.10	83.67	56.20	463.95		-15.80	86.17	-26.50	39.93	35.80
Wakefield	26.43	46.08	179.95	39.87	224.18	621.10		-12.59	77.15	59.09	-58.26	65.51
Wallasey	62.59	76.34	81.68	76.85	77.71	480.65		45.61	75.30	24.22	35.66	13.81
Walsall	49.85	295.08	93.68	84.84	94.50	699.21		17.96	98.29	94.29	27.81	71.31
Warrington	14.32	35.00	155.05	172.51	92.71	583.46		-116.45	82.85	25.69	10.04	38.88
West Bromwich	49.47	315.41	67.99	68.13	63.96	620.30		38.23	95.00	14.08	35.23	25.34
West Ham	127.79	121.37	167.55	187.75	132.53	829.45		46.20	83.46	-2.57	51.49	52.36
West Hartlepool	9.01	55.88	97.03	62.22	79.34	408.50		-936.48	88.68	85.63	-15.44	56.66
Wigan	19.47	48.83	78.47	110.30	79.87	494.27		-109.36	84.02	18.69	32.25	31.29
Wolverhampton	57.09	93.40	45.10	79.71	67.93	422.45		36.48	83.60	11.87	81.11	30.04
Worcester	1.12	65.28	65.16	97.36	64.78	416.65		25.58	70.38	-15.56	5.22	2.16
York	71.45	80.49	92.67	149.71	105.24	653.13		-5.68	64.33	46.20	-20.29	62.17
Mean	42.85	74.02	94.50	112.81	99.55	N/A		-10.75	81.41	15.76	32.14	52.07
Standard Deviation	46.86	46.59	33.90	39.11	37.75	N/A		575.57	12.20	35.74	29.30	18.38

CHAPTER THREE

Explaining Expenditure

Chapter Two dealt with a number of ways of measuring investment in municipal health services by County Boroughs during the interwar period. In particular, it demonstrated how much variety there was within the national aggregate expenditure figures, both in terms of levels of spending in individual boroughs, and in the prioritisation of different services within the overall health budget and in individual authorities. In this chapter we seek to nuance and explain this 'big picture' further by mapping out and exploring some of the more qualitative factors behind these different patterns. We introduce some of the key qualitative sources which shed light on the practices of individual boroughs, and the concerns which have emerged from them. These include the fabric of hospital buildings inherited by county boroughs in 1929; the character of the local councils; the political 'flavour' of the borough; and the nature of relations with the Ministry of Health. This also helps us to understand how and why some boroughs spent at consistently high or low levels on health over the period, while others climbed or fell down the rankings, or spent significantly more on some health services than others. Finally, we draw these approaches together to contextualise the selection of four case-study boroughs for close analysis in the subsequent chapters.

One of the most valuable sources for drilling down to see the process of local decision making is a set of Ministry of Health surveys of individual boroughs in the 1930s. These are highly detailed, yet underutilised, documents, and offer insights into a wide range of local factors which had a bearing on the provision of health care.[1] In this chapter we draw on this

1 For a rare piece of analysis which uses these sources see J. P. Bradbury, 'The 1929 Local Government Act: The Formulation and Implementation of Poor Law (Health Care) and Exchequer Grants Reform for England and Wales (Outside London)', PhD thesis, University of Bristol, 1991. See Chapter One for more details on the surveys.

series to shed light on local decision making. The surveys were not without their political agenda: they were initiated by the Ministry in order to judge the state of local authority health provision, and to assess how far councils had implemented the terms of the 1929 Local Government Act. The reports were thus partly concerned to prompt the development of particular measures (not least the development of general hospitals), but they took place within a framework of increasing constraints on spending.

The value of the reports is greatly enhanced by the fact that the Ministry inspectors generally did much more than assess the state of provision for healthcare, however; in addition, they frequently commented on the nature of obstacles to further progress; the character of the various Council committees and key officers; the state of relations with the voluntary sector; and any pertinent wider factors, such as real or perceived needs to prioritise other services. Each report also generated sometimes large amounts of correspondence between inspectors, Ministry officials, and borough representatives, and these documents give us some of the most candid information and opinions we have. In most cases the borough's subsequent progress was followed up by letter, but the worst-performing or most recalcitrant authorities were subjected to a resurvey at a later date, in order to assess how far they had taken Ministry recommendations on board. Of the seventy-nine County Boroughs in England in 1930, sixty-seven have surveys and associated documents extant (the Welsh boroughs were inspected separately by the Welsh Board of Health; a distinction to which we will return). The following sections will use the surveys and their correspondence to comment on a range of local factors affecting healthcare provision, starting with general hospitals. We will then go on to discuss what the surveys reveal about the nature of local politics (and in particular, the impact of the Labour Party) and the relationship between borough councils and the Ministry of Health.

The Appropriation of General Hospitals

We noted in Chapter Two that per capita expenditure tells only part of the story of investment in general hospitals in the years following the Local Government Act. This is partly because not all county boroughs inherited an institution at the transfer of responsibilities from the Poor Law Guardians, and those that did inherited buildings in wildly varying states of development, specialisation and design. Indeed, the variety of circumstances is such that there has until recently been no clear impression of the pattern of appropriation by county boroughs across the country. Judgements of the impact of the 1929 Act on hospital appropriation have also been variable: PEP spoke of 'revolutionary change in hospital policy' while the later commentator Sir Martin Gilbert stated that it was 'not the landmark in Poor Law history that the Webbs and other social reformers expected it would be', and other historians have supported his view (with some exceptions).[2] Assessments are frequently supported by only vague evidence, however ('some advance', 'few councils'), or are based heavily on single areas of the country.[3] Furthermore, previous discussions have tended to focus on bed numbers in appropriated institutions, rather than the question of which

2 PEP *The Hospital System. Planning Broadsheet*, 84 (London, 1934), 2, 4; B. Gilbert, *Britain Since 1918* (1967; 2nd edn, London, 1980), 62. See also, for example, S. Cherry, *Medical Services and the Hospitals in Britain, 1860–1939* (Cambridge, 1996), 5, 62; P. Thane, *Foundations of the Welfare State* (2nd edn, Harlow, 1996), 177; Fraser, *The Evolution*, 219, 234.

3 See A. Thorpe, *Britain in the 1930s* (Oxford, 1992), 111–12; M. Pugh, *'We Danced All Night': A Social History of Britain Between the Wars* (London, 2008), 55; M. Daunton, *Wealth and Welfare: An Economic and Social History of Britain 1851–1951* (Oxford, 2007), 551; M. Bruce, *The Coming of the Welfare State* (4th edn, London, 1968), 260; B. Doyle, 'The Changing Functions of Urban Government', in M. Daunton, ed., *The Cambridge Urban History of Britain*, iii: *1840–1950* (Cambridge, 2000), 29; Cherry, *Medical Services and the Hospitals*, 59; N. Timmins, *The Five Giants: A Biography of the Welfare State* (revised edn, London, 2001), 105–6; J. Pickstone, *Medicine and Industrial Society: A History of Hospital Development in Manchester and its Region, 1752–1946* (Manchester, 1985), 258–9; B. Harris, *The Origins of the British Welfare*

boroughs decided to appropriate, when and why.[4] The Ministry of Health 1930s surveys allow us to focus on this latter topic, which is vital to any understanding of what shaped municipal provision. The surveys also – vitally – allow us to map out the chronological pattern of appropriation for the first time, and this is provided in Appendix One.[5]

The unevenness of the inheritance of PAIs in 1929 is explained by the lack of correspondence between the local authority borders and those of the Poor Law Unions. Institutions which had served the poor of several authorities prior to 1929 passed to only one, and this in itself was the cause of some dispute where more than one council (sometimes including County Councils as well as County Boroughs) had designs on the institution.[6] Blackpool and Bury, for example, did not inherit an institution because it passed instead to the Lancashire County Council, while Wallasey lost out to Birkenhead County Borough. The desire to inherit an institution might correspond to ambitions in the field of welfare or healthcare, but it could just as easily relate to local urban hierarchies of function, civic pride, and long-standing competition between neighbours – all factors which are illustrated more generally in our case studies. As Appendix One shows, of the sixty-seven County Boroughs with Ministry of Health surveys extant, eight (11.9 per cent) did not inherit an institution in 1929. Such boroughs had to enter into user arrangements with County Borough or County Council neighbours, build, buy or adapt a new hospital, or rely on their existing provision.[7] Thus in the short term at least, the absence

---

State: Society, State and Social Welfare in England and Wales, 1800–1945 (Basingstoke, 2004), 232; B. B. Gilbert, *British Social Policy 1914–1939* (London, 1970), 233).

4 Examples are B. Abel-Smith, *The Hospitals 1800–1948* (London, 1964), and R. Pinker, *English Hospital Statistics 1861–1938* (London, 1966).

5 Also A. Levene, M. Powell and J. Stewart, 'The Development of Municipal General Hospitals in English County Boroughs in the 1930s', *Medical History*, 50:1 (2006),. The discussion which follows is based on the longer analysis presented in that article. The total number of hospitals with a clear date of appropriation from this source was 44, in 36 County Boroughs.

6 This point is noted for the North-West by Pickstone, *Medicine and Industrial Society*, 214.

7 Stoke, Birmingham, Coventry, Huddersfield, Hull, and Wigan all planned new hospitals in this period. Newcastle, South Shields, and Sunderland made plans to

of a transferred institution in 1930 was a constraint to the development of individual boroughs' hospital policies. Other boroughs, meanwhile, inherited several good quality institutions. This facilitated their appropriation as public general hospitals, and the development of proper separation schemes between the chronic and acute sick. Liverpool and Leeds are examples of boroughs in this category, as was the smaller borough of Hastings on the south coast.[8]

Inheriting more than one institution was a clear boon to the development of schemes for classification and thus a move towards what we might characterise as an ongoing hospital *policy*. Of course, these boroughs also tended to be the larger authorities, which also often attracted the more progressive and ambitious health officers (most notably the Medical Officers of Health), and tended to have above-average levels of income from the rates. However, inheriting an institution did not automatically make it suitable for medical rather than welfare purposes. The survey documents make it clear that for the boroughs which inherited only one institution, the state and nature of the building was very significant in this respect. In some cases, the institution was simply not suitable for development as a general hospital: the infirmary might be part of the mixed workhouse, or the two might share facilities such as laundries and kitchens which would make separation very difficult. The Feetham Institute in Darlington was a mixed one (both workhouse and Poor Law infirmary), with parts of each half lying on either side of a road. The infirmary had been developed piecemeal, and was hard to nurse. The Ministry's surveyor judged that 'the Medical Officer of Health is very wise to advise his Council not to sink

build or expand which were halted by the outbreak of war. M. Powell, 'An Expanding Service: Municipal Acute Medicine in the 1930s', *Twentieth Century British History*, 8:3 (1997), 343.

8 See A. Levene, 'Between Less Eligibility and the NHS: The Changing Place of Poor Law Hospitals in England and Wales, 1929–39', *Twentieth Century British History* (2009); TNA MH66/665, Ministry of Health Survey Report (hereafter all this series' reports are referred to as Survey Report), Hastings. The Hastings and East Sussex councils had evolved a scheme whereby the sick from both councils were to be accommodated in the Hastings institution, which could then be appropriated. The scheme was shelved by 1934, however and not resurrected.

much capital in it'.[9] In Hastings, the infirmary and workhouse parts of the PAI were 'so inextricably mixed that separation would be impossible without incurring an unjustifiable expense.'[10] Other buildings were outdated, crowded, and unfeasibly expensive to equip for modern medicine and surgery. In 1946 Aneurin Bevan called the worst of these institutions, 'monstrous buildings, a cross between a workhouse and a barracks – or a prison.'[11] In these cases it was sometimes deemed more appropriate, by both council and Ministry, to simply build a new general hospital. Lincoln's Burton Road PAI, for example, was described by the surveyor as 'the least satisfactory Poor Law Infirmary which I have yet encountered in a County Borough.' Ward floors were uneven and nursing was made difficult by small spaces between beds. Some wards had radiators projecting into them, along the length of patients' beds. All the wards were overcrowded, and there was no proper classification. The appropriation of this institution was not recommended, highlighting the fact that it was not automatically assumed to be the best course of action by the Ministry.[12]

The number and state of the inherited buildings, therefore, dictated to a certain extent what could be done with them. The Ministry's Annual Report for 1930–1 noted that the boroughs with separate Poor Law infirmaries had generally appropriated them rapidly after 1929, and that the difficulty of separation from the workhouse proved the main obstacle to appropriation elsewhere (see Figure 3.1).[13] In total, 39 per cent of appropriations made by the end of the interwar period had taken place in 1930, and another 9 per cent in 1931. By 1936, thirty-seven boroughs had appropriated at least one general hospital. However, the survey reports indicate that a wide range of less easily measurable factors also played a part in the decision to appropriate (or not) and to invest further.

9 TNA MH66/571, Survey Report, Darlington.
10 TNA MH66/665, Survey Report, Hastings.
11 Aneurin Bevan, Hansard, House of Commons, 30 April 1946, 422, cols 48–9.
12 TNA MH66/718, Survey Report, Lincoln.
13 Ministry of Health Annual Report, 1930–1, 51–2.

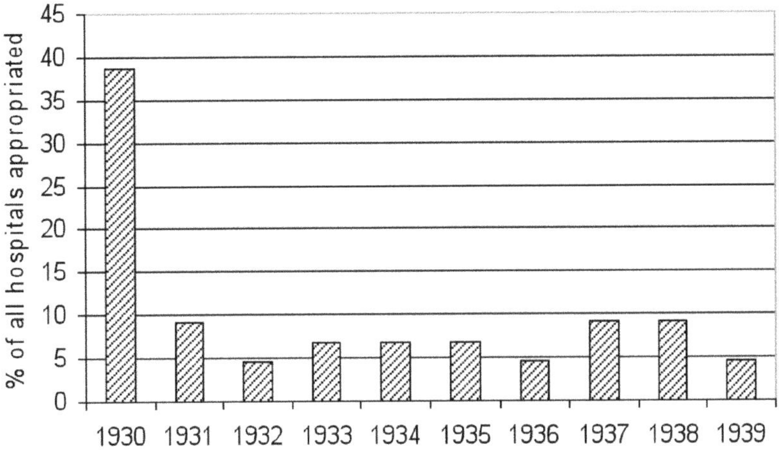

Figure 3.1 The Pace of Hospital Appropriation, 1930–9
Sources: Ministry of Health County Borough Surveys, 1930–9, TNA MH66 419–1023. The total number of hospitals with a clear date of appropriation from this source was forty-four.

One of the principal reasons offered by boroughs unwilling to invest in their transferred institution was that it was too expensive. The Ministry was often unsympathetic to this attitude, stating that appropriation should not in itself bring increased costs (the principal factor cited by local councils against it), and that it was in any case important enough to be a priority. Some boroughs arguing this position really were poorly off in terms of rate income: Barnsley, Bolton and Burton-on-Trent, for example, all also spent at below average levels on other health services. This situation only worsened for many authorities as the Depression took hold. Some of the north-eastern Boroughs were granted 'Special Areas' status from the mid-1930s on the grounds of their depressed economic situation, giving them particularly legitimate grounds for parsimony – and the Ministry recognised this.[14] Authorities elsewhere in the country were also struggling with heavy burdens

14 This label was attached to certain areas by the Depressed Areas Bill of November 1934. W. R. Garside, *British Unemployment, 1919–39* (Cambridge, 1990), 255. See also Levene *et al.*, 'The Development of Municipal General Hospitals'.

of unemployment and economic slump. Even affluent and high-spending Eastbourne made the same argument about the costs of appropriation, however, indicating that it was not straightforwardly linked to income, or to expenditure on health more broadly.[15] Sometimes a borough pleaded other commitments which prevented investment in a hospital: Gloucester and Blackpool cited the need to keep rates down in defence of their reluctance to spend, for example, while Bournemouth council apparently did not feel that their town needed further investment in health.[16] The Ministry often detected apathy in these pleas, however, stating of Burton-on-Trent that 'the arguments against appropriation are those almost universally employed by Councils who have no intention of improving their hospital services.'[17]

In other cases, the survey documents indicate that a desire to expand health services, civic pride and/or the zeal of one or two officers led to the opposite charge: that of excessive extravagance. This not infrequently emerged after a council had dragged its feet over improving a transferred institution, and then produced a lavish scheme to build a new hospital instead. Doncaster, for example, had protested against the appropriation of Springwell House, but then approved a plan for a new hospital costing £100,000.[18] Given that the local County Council was also building a new hospital, the Ministry was not happy to sanction a loan for capital expenditure until active co-operation with this authority and the voluntary hospitals had been ruled out. Springwell House was ultimately not appropriated; nor does a new hospital seem to have been built by the time of a post-war survey by the Ministry of Health and Nuffield Hospital Trust.

15 TNA MH66/1066, Survey Report, Barnsley; TNA MH66/459 Survey Report, Bolton; TNA MH66/507, Resurvey Correspondence, Burton; TNA MH66/596, Survey Correspondence, Eastbourne.

16 TNA MH66/473, Survey Report, Bournemouth. The surveyor's response in his report was that 'the town is not so exceptional that it can afford to neglect its Public Health services'.

17 TNA MH66/625, 454 and 473, Survey Reports, Gloucester, Blackpool and Bournemouth; TNA MH66/507, Resurvey Correspondence, Burton-on-Trent. The Blackpool council did point out that as a resort town, much of their commercial income was concentrated in three months of the year. This may have led to a cautious attitude towards finance, although they were by no means the only borough in this position.

18 TNA MH66/584, Survey Report, Doncaster.

The inspectors did not find only gloomy scenarios; some boroughs adopted the need to integrate hospital development into their wider health schemes with apparently little debate. Bradford and Croydon, for example, were both singled out for praise: they had several institutions available, a progressive attitude to health care already evident, and energetic people in key posts to press for further reform. Welshman, Pickstone and Steven Cherry have highlighted other examples of developing municipal hospital sectors in individual County Boroughs.[19] In other cases, a variety of local antagonisms and personality clashes held things up. This was frequently based on ill feeling between the Public Health and PACs, with the latter protective of the institutions they had inherited from the Poor Law, and unwilling to let them pass into other hands. This was exacerbated when the members of the PAC had previously been Poor Law Guardians, and so had a long relationship with the institution. It was said of Stockport that '[t]he Local Government Act is a dead letter; the old Guardians still reign supreme.'[20] In the least-delicately handled cases this might lead to the MOH being excluded from the transferred institution, as we will see happened in the case study town of Barnsley.[21] The Ministry tended to be

19 J. Welshman, *Municipal Medicine: Public Health in Twentieth Century Britain* (Bern, 2000); Pickstone, *Medicine and Industrial Society*, 274; S. Cherry, 'Regional Comparators in the Funding and Organization of the Voluntary Hospital System, c. 1860–1939' in M. Gorsky and S. Sheard, eds, *Financing Medicine: The British Experience since 1750* (London, 2006), 71.

20 TNA, MH66/898, Survey Report, Stockport.

21 N. Wilson, *Municipal Health Services* (London, 1946), 170–1. C. Webster, *The Health Services since the War*, i: *Problems of Health Care – The National Health Service before 1957* (London, 1988), 8, notes the role of the MOH in setting the standards of municipal health care generally. J. Lewis, *What Price Community Medicine? The Philosophy, Practice and Politics of Public Health Since 1919* (Brighton, 1986), also highlights the increased profile of MOHs up to the interwar period. This tension between councils was exacerbated when the PAC was made up of ex-Poor Law Guardians, who might have considerable pride invested in the more modern PACs. J. M. Mackintosh, *Trends of Opinion about the Public Health, 1901–51* (Oxford, 1953), 132, wrote in the 1950s that 'it is difficult to overestimate the enthusiasm with which the new Public Assistance Committees set about their task of transforming the old institutions and reclassifying their inmates.' This picture is not borne out by

somewhat exasperated at this disinclination to see council expenditure as coming from one purse, but it was a significant and recurring brake on expansion.[22]

One of the greatest potential spurs to a developed plan for health care was an active and energetic MOH. In Bristol the MOH was said to be a man of ingenuity and diplomacy, who had the courage to face opposition.[23] In Manchester, Dr Veitch Clark (who later contributed to the Ministry/Nuffield post-war survey of hospital provision) spearheaded improvements in health care.[24] In Doncaster, however, this officer was an elderly man who had 'exercised an excessive zeal for economy'.[25] Generally, the reports show MOHs claiming to be in favour of appropriation, and where these officers were both dynamic and diplomatic *and* had the support of the council, they were often able to exert a significant influence on decision making. In other cases, personal weakness, and intransigent opposition left MOHs unable or unwilling to fight their corner.

Appropriation in itself did not necessarily mean continued investment or improved standards, however, as Powell has noted.[26] Here, ongoing expenditure patterns can be usefully joined up with the picture created from the survey reports to examine how appropriation translated into ongoing hospital policy. These figures show that the boroughs which appropriated hospitals fell into two groups. First, there were those which showed a steady level of investment in general hospitals after appropriation. Second, there were those which showed peaks of investment in certain years. Within

---

the Ministry Surveys however, although they of course had an interest in removing the hospitals from the PACs in favour of the PHCs.

22 The Minister of Health noted this tendency in his Annual Report for 1932–3, 'of [councils] regarding particular problems as the problems only of a single committee'. Ministry of Health Annual Report, 1932–3, p. 35.

23 TNA, MH66/584, Survey Report, Doncaster.

24 TNA, MH66/487, Survey Report, Bristol; Pickstone, *Medicine and Industrial Society*, 259. In London, also, the centralising role of the County MOH has been noted in the success of the hospital provisions of the Local Government Act : J. Stewart, '"For a healthy London": The Socialist Medical Association and the London County Council in the 1930s', *Medical History*, 41:4 (1997).

25 TNA MH66/584, Survey Report, Doncaster.

26 Powell, 'An Expanding Service', 345.

these groups, however, there was also variation, as illustrated in Figure 3.2. Of twenty-nine boroughs with at least three years' data on hospital expenditure by 1936–7, eight continued to spend at a steady but low level on their hospitals (represented in the figure by the West Midlands borough of Coventry); while four others did not particularly increase their expenditure on hospitals over the period, but were steady, high investors (represented by Halifax, in West Yorkshire). These trends probably at least partly reflect the state of the individual hospital, but they also speak of different attitudes to hospital *policy*. The boroughs which increased their expenditure on hospitals over the 1930s also show different patterns of investment. Among this group, about a third made a cash injection in the year after appropriation, a third did so several years after appropriation, and a third increased their expenditure as part of a steadily increasing trend over several years. These different patterns are represented by Derby, Liverpool and Manchester, respectively. This again suggests a variety of responses to hospital development – a rapid response to the change; a delayed reaction perhaps based on financial constraints; and an ongoing movement which took on momentum over time.

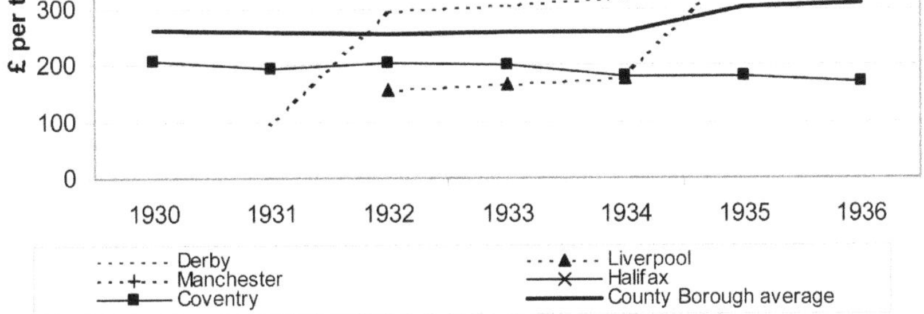

Figure 3.2 Expenditure per Thousand on General Hospitals by Selected County Boroughs, 1930–6
Source: Local Government Financial Statistics, 1930–6

It is equally instructive to consider the course of capital expenditure, which will capture investment in building stock and equipment, and thus perhaps more accurately reflect the investment needed to update hospital buildings after the transfer to public health. This must, however, be placed in the context of curtailed Ministry sanction for expenditure in the difficult 1930s.[27] Figure 3.3 shows the capital expenditure figures per thousand for the same boroughs as were shown in the earlier figure. The two boroughs representing steady spenders (Halifax and Coventry) both invested more in capital projects early in the period than their constant level of revenue expenditure would suggest, and were either at or above the County Borough average. It is possible, however, that these boroughs were committed to capital outlay under the Poor Law, which the PHC merely took over. Since the capital investment did not bring increased revenue expense, we may speculate that it consisted of improvements to wards or equipment rather than new buildings, which would bring increased lighting, heating and staff costs. The steady revenue expenditure may therefore mask significant outlay in terms of capital, a fact which is particularly notable in the case of Coventry, which spent at a low level.

The boroughs which showed an upward pattern of investment from the revenue account did tend to match this in capital outlay. Derby, the early investor, seems to have undertaken two capital projects, in 1931 and 1933. This suggests a rapid commitment to development and improvement, although it may also indicate that the buildings inherited by this borough were in a very poor condition, necessitating heavy investment. Liverpool and Manchester also matched their revenue expenditure with capital outlay. Liverpool spent at a higher level from the capital account in 1935, although not on the scale of Derby; the same year that it showed a rise in revenue expenditure. It should be borne in mind, however, that Liverpool had several institutions while Derby did not, making the latter's capital outlay the more notable. Manchester too spent at a raised level on capital projects in the last years of the period, as they did out of rate income, although the level was not very high.

27 Some boroughs were placed on Ministry blacklists for loan sanctions, depending on their financial situation. See S. V. Ward, 'Implementation Versus Planmaking: the Example of List Q and the Depressed Areas 1922–39', *Planning Perspectives*, 1 (1986).

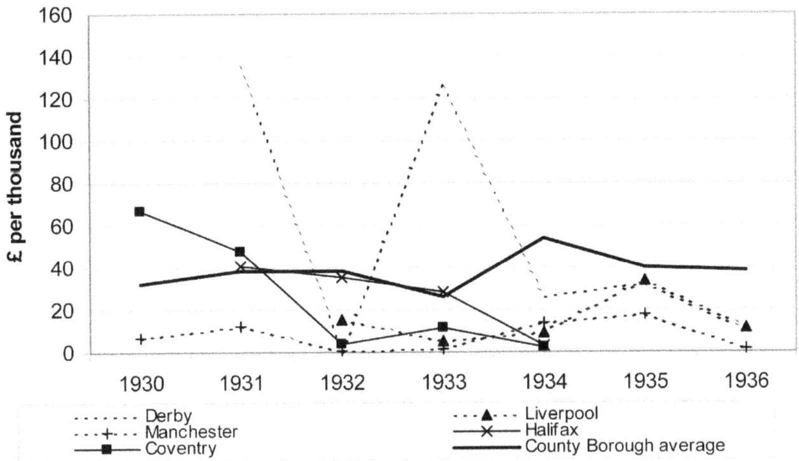

Figure 3.3 Capital Investment on General Hospitals in Selected County Boroughs, 1930–6
Source: Local Government Financial Statistics, 1930–6

Generally, therefore, the boroughs which showed a rise in revenue expenditure showed a matching rise in capital projects. Even those boroughs which spent at a steadier level, however, occasionally did still commit themselves to capital development. The lack of a corresponding rise in revenue expenditure suggests that it was on improvements to existing facilities rather than new wards and buildings, which would have brought increased revenue costs. The expenditure data do, therefore, suggest a variation in the continued policy towards appropriated hospital buildings in different boroughs – from those which maintained a consistent level of spending, while perhaps also investing in capital, to those which were more energetic in their policy. Again, much probably depended on the need for capital investment when the hospital was handed over from the PAC, as well as council attitudes.

The survey reports and correspondence set alongside the expenditure data, thus highlight a range of local factors which were significant in explaining appropriation and subsequent investment patterns. Many of these factors are not easy to quantify and are missed in investigations based solely on expenditure or bed data. The character of individuals like the MOH, the Town Clerk or the Council Treasurer, for example, could have a disproportionate but non-quantifiable impact on health policy.[28] This is borne out when the impact of some of those factors which *can* be measured in some way is measured: only population size had much effect on the likelihood that a borough with a transferred institution would appropriate it.[29] Appropriating boroughs also had small voluntary sectors – a topic which there is not space to explore here, but which will be investigated in greater detail in the case-study chapters – and also tended to be relatively high spenders on other health services. The influence of overtly political factors played little part when measured quantitatively, in contrast with the emphasis placed on individuals in the surveys. The next section will investigate this area in greater detail.

Local Politics and the Role of the Labour Party

The influence of overtly political factors is diluted by the suggestion that local politics prior to the interwar period were not, generally speaking, party politics in the way that we think of them today. Instead, local councillors have been characterised as focusing primarily on keeping the rates down, with little sense of individuals acting along party lines. This is not to suggest that local politics were consensual, but there is some agreement that it took the increased presence of the Parliamentary Labour Party in Parliament after the First World War to inject national politics into the local arena, and to prompt the non-socialist parties to define themselves in clearer

28 This is also noted by E. H. Rhodes, 'Personality in Public Administration', *Journal of Public Administration*, 8:3 (1930), 250–2.

29 Larger boroughs were more likely to appropriate. This was linked to the likelihood that large boroughs inherited more than one institution, but had a separate (and stronger) impact in its own right. See Levene *et al.*, 'The Development of Municipal General Hospitals' for details of the variables used, and the method.

terms as well. Others, however, criticise this view as being overly simplistic, stating that party politics had long been present in local government, but that Labour did perhaps energise it, and stimulate other parties to organise along more well prescribed lines.[30] Nonetheless, it is the Labour Party which has remained particularly emblematic of the development of local party politics, and also with raised levels of investment in the local arena.

One reason for this was that Labour had a well defined sense of identity even at the local level. It had had its first successes in local government, which was more accessible than the national scene, and also required less capital investment.[31] Labour had appointed an Advisory Committee on Local Government at the end of the First World War, and it provided financial support for its candidates at the local level. In return, however, it expected them to represent the party view in council: failure to toe the party line in public could lead to loss of the whip.[32] In the early 1920s, the national party also issued local government manifestoes, handbooks of local government, and broadcast eve of poll addresses, all in an attempt to raise consciousness of the party, and spread its identity.[33] This level of organisation had not been seen in the other parties, and was frequently resented by them for taking local matters out of local hands. However, by the end of the interwar period, subjects for debate in council had frequently been discussed by several of the party caucuses prior to the council meetings.[34] This is an example of early Labour organisation in local politics, and the way that it subsequently spurred other parties to define themselves and adopt party lines. However, as we will see in our case studies, not all Labour parties were the same; nor were their opponents a homogenous group.

30 B. Keith-Lucas and P. G. Richards, *A History of Local Government in the Twentieth Century* (London, 1978), 114–15; J. Rowett, 'The Labour Party and Local Government: Theory and Practice in the Interwar Years', DPhil thesis, University of Oxford, 1979, 1–2; J. G. Bulpitt, *Party Politics in English Local Government* (London, 1967), 1–7.

31 A. L. Beach, 'The Labour Party and the Idea of Citizenship, c.1931–1951', PhD thesis, University of London, 1996, 130. See also M. Worley, *Labour Inside the Gate: a History of the British Labour Party Between the Wars* (London, 2005), 154, 197.

32 Keith-Lucas and Richards, *A History of Local Government*, 119–20 and 130.

33 Rowett 'The Labour Party', 31–4.

34 Keith-Lucas and Richards, *A History of Local Government*, 130.

There is also a tendency to equate Labour with spending and levelling, because of its commitment to working-class health and welfare. This association, together with the contemporary concerns that surrounded the party in some areas, can lead to a simplistic assumption that socialism equalled 'progressive' policies, particularly in areas like health. Certainly the Labour Party has been studied in these terms in much of the literature on politics and municipal services, but with the exception of Powell's 1995 work, this has all focused on the post-war period, when the degree of local determinism in budget setting was significantly different from the interwar years.[35] In one such study L. J. Sharpe and K. Newton note the commonly accepted paradigm that Labour was inclined to spend more than right-of-centre parties, but correctly state that it may not necessarily have held true for all services: the right might favour investment where productivity or growth was enhanced, and their mainly middle-class supporters may have supported expenditure on areas such as secondary education.[36] The more pertinent question for the current study is how far Labour was inclined to

35 M. Powell, 'Did Politics Matter? Municipal Health Expenditure in the 1930s', *Urban History*, 22:3 (1995). The most prominent difference is the centralisation of budget setting after 1948.

36 L. J. Sharpe and K. Newton, *Does Politics Matter? The Determinants of Public Policy* (Oxford, 1984), 14. In fact, these authors state that Labour boroughs in the 1960s and 1970s did spend more highly on redistributive and socially ameliorative services such as housing, education and health. T. Hansen, 'Transforming Needs into Expenditure Decisions', in K. Newton and F. Pinter, eds, *Urban Political Economy* (London, 1981), 41, also suggests that non-socialists may spend highly because they prioritise costly individual solutions. See also J. E. Alt, 'Some Social and Political Correlates of County Borough Expenditures', *British Journal of Political Science*, 1 (1971); F. R. Oliver and J. Stanyer, 'Some Aspects of the Financial Behaviour of County Boroughs', *Public Administration*, 47 (1969); D. N. King, 'Why do Local Authority Rate Poundages Differ?', *Public Administration*, 51 (1973). L. Marks, *Metropolitan Maternity: Maternity and Infant Welfare Services in Early Twentieth-Century London* (Amsterdam, 1996), found that Labour strength in the Metropolitan Boroughs of Woolwich and Stepney was 'a key factor determining their high levels of expenditure on municipal provision for maternal and child welfare' (p. 64). S. V. Ward (*The Geography of Interwar Britain: The State and Uneven Development* (London, 1988), 201) however, has suggested that although Labour may have been inclined

spend highly *per se* and how far this interacted with the socio-economic characteristics of the boroughs they had influence in. In particular, the party tended to have a higher profile in poorer areas with low rateable values and high levels of need, meaning that they needed to set higher rates in the pound in order to spend even at the national average.[37] There does however, appear to be a certain amount of consensus around the fact that in England and Wales, the Labour Party did spend more highly than non-Socialist parties on ameliorative and redistributive policies, of which public health was one.

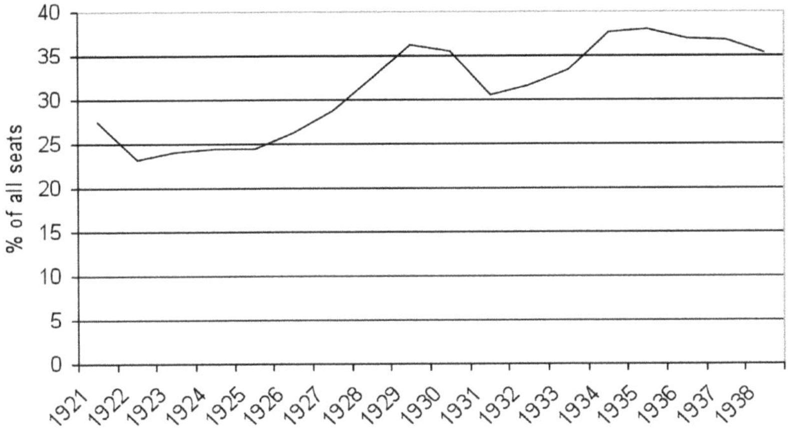

Figure 3.4 Proportion of County Borough Seats Held by Labour in Interwar England and Wales
Source: *The Times*, annual municipal election returns, 1922–36.
See Note 34 for further details on the data

to spend highly, they could exercise little discretion in this direction in the case of a really poor borough such as Gateshead.

37 Alt, 'Some Social and Political Correlates', 54–5; Oliver and Stanyer, 'Some Aspects', 177–8; King 'Why do Local Authority Rate Poundages Differ?', 168–72; Sharpe and Newton, *Does Politics Matter?*, 205; Hansen, 'Transforming Needs', 27–47.

The Ministry of Health surveys, together with election returns and contemporary newspaper reporting, reveal that the Labour Party was seen in many of the same terms during the interwar period as well, although its direct impact on local policies varied greatly. This was the period of many of Labour's first council majorities, and thus their first opportunity to have much of an impact on decision making. Figure 3.4 shows the growth of Labour representation over the interwar period for those county boroughs whose election returns were reported in *The Times*.[38] In 1913, Labour held around 400 out of 7000 seats on County Borough councils, although their strength and activism had distinct regional features: in Lancashire and Yorkshire, for example, around half of all seats were contested by the party, while elsewhere very few candidates were fielded.[39] On average, Labour held 25 per cent of all council seats from 1922 to 1926, perhaps finding it hard to break through strengthening anti-Socialist pacts. In the 1926 local elections the party gained 153 seats, concentrated in the northern and midland mining and industrial areas, and won control of Sheffield, the first Labour-controlled city in the country.[40] The proportion of Labour

38 The returns were published after the municipal elections in November of each year. In any one year, one third of the council seats became available for re-election, which may have made a swing in political opinion slower to appear than in the County Councils, where the whole council was re-elected every year. There is also a degree of uncertainty surrounding the returns for the earlier years of the period, when the newspaper reported the change in seats from the previous year, rather than stating the composition of the new council, as it started to do from 1928. Since Labour candidates generally consistently identified themselves as such, however, any uncertainty as to Labour representation is minimised. There were several boroughs whose results were never reported in *The Times*, but this number fell over the period, from 20 in 1922 to 12 in 1930. The missing boroughs had a significant positive correlation with wealth (rateable value), at 0.448, which was significant at a 99 per cent level of confidence. Other evidence on wealth and politics suggests that these missing boroughs were unlikely to have been Labour strongholds, and that the results should not therefore be greatly affected by their absence, although we would ideally prefer to have a complete set of data.

39 Rowett, 'The Labour Party', 4.

40 Ibid. 15. Rowett also notes the fact that Labour was in this year allied to the national mining dispute, which may have increased support (16).

seats then began to rise, reaching 36 per cent in 1929. There were reversals in the elections of 1930 and 1931, when *The Times* noted the loss of Derby, Stoke and Birkenhead, under the headline 'Labour defeat'. Not one of the twenty-four Labour candidates at Birmingham was returned in 1931, and Labour lost 206 seats to its five gains, in the face of more disciplined Liberal/Conservative alliances.[41] In 1933, however, there were significant gains for Labour, retaking Barrow, Norwich, Sheffield and Swansea, and winning Bootle and Lincoln for the first time.[42] Thereafter, the average proportion of seats held returned to around 30–35 per cent. By 1939 it had majorities in eighteen County Boroughs, although John Rowett suggests that it had reached a plateau of support both locally and nationally.[43] In some boroughs, Labour was never a strong force: in Burton-on-Trent and Portsmouth, for example, it never gained more than 15 per cent of council seats, while in Labour strongholds such as Merthyr and West Ham, the party averaged 71 per cent of seats over the period. Labour had particular success in the East End of London and the East Midlands, and in the heavy industrial areas of Lancashire, South Yorkshire and South Wales, where they campaigned for benefits for the unemployed.[44]

Whatever the level of party organisation in County Borough councils, what does seem to be undisputed is that other parties perceived Labour as a threat, and began to form alliances to keep them out of local government.[45] It is difficult to determine the extent of this development, as coalitions are not always identified as such in national election reports, but there were certainly groups of councillors identifying themselves as Citizens in Sheffield, the Municipal Alliance in West Ham, Anti-Labour in Reading

41 *The Times*, 02 November 1931, Rowett, 'The Labour Party', 234.

42 Rowett, 'The Labour Party', 236.

43 Keith-Lucas and Richards, *A History of Local Government*, 113–14, Rowett, 'The Labour Party', 241 and 252.

44 Rowett, 'The Labour Party', 22.

45 This phenomenon is one of the three main developments in local politics identified by Cook from 1918 to 1928, along with the rise of the Labour challenge, and the decline of the Liberals. C. Cook, 'Liberals, Labour and Local Elections', in G. Peale and C. Cook, eds, *The Politics of Reappraisal, 1918–1938* (London, 1975), 167.

and Doncaster, and Ratepayers in Croydon and East Ham over the course of the period.[46] Other councillors returned simply as Liberal or Conservative may have made arrangements to avoid three-cornered fights in order to keep Labour out.[47]

This threat was generally based on an opinion which was held by many contemporary critics, namely that the party's primary characteristic was a well developed inclination to spend money, and hence raise local rates. The pejorative overtones attached to the party label in the context of local politics are clear in several contemporary sources, including the coverage of municipal elections in *The Times*. In 1930, the newspaper described Socialists as 'those who are ..., by their political faith, devoted to extravagance rather than retrenchment'.[48] Under a headline of 'The Socialist Menace', the newspaper urged in 1926 that 'the utmost vigilance on the part of [Labour's] opponents will be necessary if the Socialist attack is to be defeated.'[49] And in 1932, the anti-Labour sentiment was again made clear: 'if apathy can be dispelled there is an excellent opportunity to-day [polling day] to bring about a further substantial reduction in the Socialist strength on many important councils.'[50] Members of the Labour Party attempted to distance themselves from this association by considering alternatives to the rating system, trying to avoid an inevitable anti-Socialist backlash if heavy demands on local purses did lead to rate increases.[51] It is clear nonetheless that some sections of society, at least, believed that extravagance was a byword for Labour, and that this threatened the status quo.

Several health surveys in the 1930s reported the same point of view. A Ministry surveyor in Bournemouth, for example, was told in confidence by the chairman of the Public Health Committee in relation to the question

46 *The Times*, municipal election reports, 1922–36.

47 Keith-Lucas and Richards (*A History of Local Government*, 114–15) cites examples of pacts of this type in English county boroughs.

48 *The Times*, 01 November 1930.

49 *The Times*, 01 November 1926.

50 *The Times*, 01 November 1932.

51 Beach, 'The Labour Party and the Idea of Citizenship', 156. No satisfactory alternative to the rates was found, although the party for a while favoured a tax on land values.

of appropriation (which was associated with increased spending in many minds, as noted above), 'that the question was erroneously regarded as purely political and the overwhelmingly conservative majority looked upon appropriation as a socialist measure which should be opposed.'[52] The survey report for Derby also used these terms of reference although this time in a more positive way; the surveyor reporting that the borough council had until recently performed poorly in the field of health provision, but that more recently, and 'probably as a result of the gradually increasing power of a Labour majority on the Council ... they ha[d] commenced to come forward and develop along lines which if continued should bring them into the front rank as a health authority.'[53] Perhaps significantly, a handwritten note from a Ministry official next to this comment says 'omit all references as to politics'. *The Times* was less restrained, reporting in 1930 that the central Labour Party had 'exercised remorseless pressure on local authorities to undertake fresh expenditure.'[54] The Ministry, however, generally made little of specific parties in its reports, and instead was inclined to look to infighting between council members and committees to explain spending levels.

Even where they were not regarded as an explicit threat by others on the council, Labour representatives were often seen as pandering only to the interests of their class: in Newport, following the repeated defeat of a water improvement scheme the local newspaper characterised its opponents as being 'largely sectional and selfish':

> the Labour Party held (we believe wrongly) that it would be impossible to provide municipal houses for the working classes and municipal water for the community as a whole, so they preferred to oppose the larger scheme, preferring to serve (as they thought) the interests of their class.[55]

52 TNA MH66/476, Survey Correspondence, Bournemouth.

53 TNA MH66/577, Survey Report, Derby.

54 *The Times*, 01 November 1930.

55 'The Talybont Poll', *South Wales Argus*, 24 January 1920.

Some Labour councillors did act in ways which supported this suspicion, by vocally advocating measures which would improve opportunities for the poor and the unemployed. This often did involve increased expenditure, for example on unemployment relief. Some Labour councils – such as Sheffield – were noted to offer larger than average unemployment relief payments, and to refuse only a small proportion of applications for interim relief in the 1930s.[56] This commitment to assisting the poor also led to Labour opposition to the 1929 Local Government Act because of a belief that it did not represent a real commitment to assist necessitous areas.[57] The Labour MP Arthur Greenwood, who became Minister of Health in the 1929 Labour administration, moved an amendment to refuse a second reading of the Bill, which he felt perpetuated the evils of the Poor law, 'fail[ed] to make unemployment a national responsibility, and [would] not appreciably relieve the financial position of necessitous areas.'[58] Comments such as this from a high-profile Labour MP inevitably drew attention to the party's desire to invest in ameliorative policies, which was coupled with an undertone of mistrust that such a comparatively new party could be trusted with wider issues.

Contemporary opinion at both national and local level thus supports the idea that the Labour Party was being singled out as having distinctive plans for expenditure. We can measure the impact of this attitude on health expenditure by returning briefly to the national aggregate figures. Figure 3.5 shows average expenditure per thousand population by boroughs with

56 Ward, *The Geography of Interwar Britain*, 144, notes that while this may have been partly related to differences in circumstances, Labour councils were also perceived as being more 'soft'; Rowett, 'The Labour Party', 307, states that in 1931, the Labour stronghold of Sheffield allowed 67.2 percent of applications and renewals for unemployment payments at the maximum rate, and disallowed only 4.9 percent, compared to 19.6 percent at maximum rates in Liverpool, and 22.3 percent disallowed in Birmingham.

57 Rowett, 'The Labour Party', 155–60, notes these criticisms also, which were based on the belief that the principle motivation for grant reform was merely to fill the financial gap left by the de-rating measures, and an eleventh-hour attempt to gain political advantage.

58 *Parliamentary Debates*, Official report, fifth series, House of Commons, 1928–9, Vol. 223 (London, 1929), cols 108–120.

a consistently low proportion of Labour councillors (always under 20 per cent) compared with those with a high level of Labour representation (always over 30 per cent, and showing a majority at some point over the period). There is a clear indication that Labour-dominated boroughs spent more on average, and that the difference became more pronounced over the period. This trend suggests that socialism, at least on this straightforward measure, did equate with raised spending levels on health.

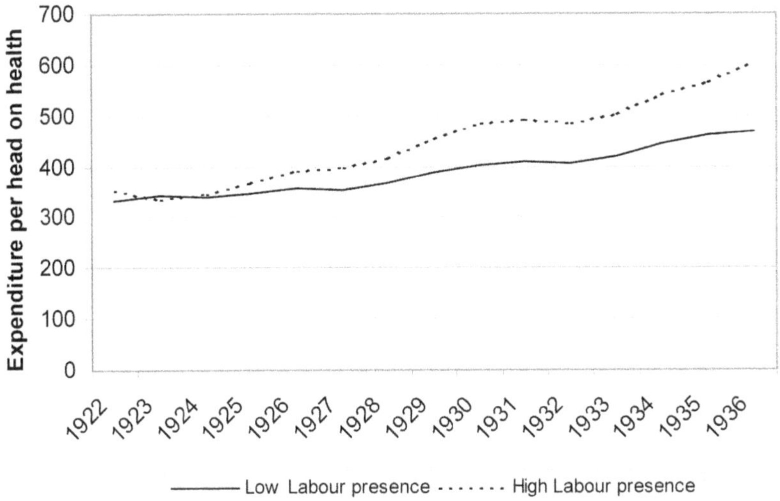

Figure 3.5 Expenditure per Head on Health in High and Low Labour Boroughs, 1922–36
Source: Local Government Financial Statistics, 1922–36, *The Times*, municipal election results, 1922–36.
There were sixteen low Labour and twenty high Labour boroughs. See text for definitions of high and low Labour.

A more penetrating analysis can be carried out by using correlation and regression analysis to investigate precisely what factors were associated with raised expenditure in Labour-influenced areas. Studies using correlation analysis, which tests the strength of association between different variables, has found that local authorities with a high proportion of Labour councillors tended also to have high social and economic needs.[59] This is true for the interwar dataset as well: using information from Registrar General and census reports we find that, in general, Labour areas had young populations and large families (both indicators of high dependency ratios); high infant mortality rates (associated with poor standards of living generally); a large proportion of miners among the male workforce and relatively high male unemployment (signs of economic depression); and an even sex ratio, or one skewed slightly in favour of males (female dominated areas tended to be relatively affluent ones, with a high rates of domestic service).[60] Labour areas also had a strong tendency to have low rateable values (indicating that the size and quality of the housing stock on which the rates were based was not high), high rates in the pound, and there was a clear association with the level of block grant received after 1930. This was designed to be responsive to local needs, so this is a further confirmation that Labour areas tended to have high socio-economic (and by implication, healthcare) needs.[61] High rates correlate with indicators of poverty, but also with high levels of expenditure on health.

These results thus return us to the question brought out in similar studies for the post-war period: were high rates in Labour areas the result of a low base rate of income (poor resources), or of an inclination to spend highly on council services? Significantly, there was an increasingly strong positive correlation between Labour representation and expenditure on health over the period – excluding that on general hospitals. This is almost certainly because of the range of non-political factors which were significant in setting hospital policy, as noted above. However, the general

59 Rowett, 'The Labour Party', 284; Alt, 'Some Social and Political Correlates'.

60 There were also significant positive correlations between Labour influence and population size in some years.

61 The needs indicators used in the calculation of the block grant were unemployment, the proportion of children under the age of five, and financial resources. See Wilson, *Municipal Health Services* (n. 23), 148–9. There was no significant association between Labour and the amount of percentage health grant received up to 1929 (whereby the government matched a proportion of expenditure on certain services); but we have seen that the proportion of Labour seats was still low in aggregate at this time.

correspondence between Labour and spending on health confirms the association in the literature between socialism and personal healthcare, and that this trend was a growing one.

We can move closer to understanding the *nature* of the relationship between Labour, needs, and expenditure, by moving from correlation to regression analysis. This measures the *impact* of one variable – or an array of variables – on another, rather than simply its coexistence.[62] In this case, the effect is measured of needs (the infant mortality rate), resources (rateable value and grant income) and Labour (percentage of council seats), on expenditure on personal health services. A different model was created for each year of the interwar period, in order to examine whether the strength and direction of any associations changed over time.[63] Modelled alone, high Labour representation had a positive effect on total expenditure, and on the major services (TB and MCW) in many years, and one which strengthened over time – but it took on more explanatory power when it was modelled in combination with other variables.[64] This suggests that Labour *per se* was not enough to promote higher expenditure; it needed other characteristics to have a significant impact. One of these was wealth, which suggests that while Labour boroughs were always inclined to spend highly on health, in the earlier years of the period in particular, they were

62 When multivariate analysis is carried out, the effect of the other measures in the model is held constant – that is, any interaction between variables will not be measured twice. The framework adopted is of the output study, measuring the effects of needs, resources and disposition on expenditure levels. Sharpe and Newton, *Does Politics Matter?*; Powell, 'Did Politics Matter?'; G. A. Boyne, *Constraints, Choices and Public Policies* (Greenwich, Conn., 1996).

63 The amount of variance in expenditure which can be explained by these models is relatively high for the first half of the period (40–50 per cent), though falling somewhat thereafter (to a low of 15 per cent in 1934). It still compares favourably with those produced by other studies. Sharpe and Newton for example, explain approximately 20 percent of variance in expenditure on personal health services. The higher amount of explanation achieved here may be partly because the decision making processes were concentrated in the local rather than the central arena in the interwar period. Sharpe and Newton, *Does Politics Matter?*, 110.

64 That is, it showed higher p-values.

only able to do so when resources were relatively high. Correlation analysis has shown, however, that Labour was unlikely to coexist with wealth in the same borough. As time went on, and Labour consolidated and increased their position, the political variable came to be a powerful causative factor in its own right. The IMR, representing needs, was rarely statistically significant, and the relationship is of high needs and *low* expenditure. This suggests that areas with high needs were not able to afford to spend highly, perhaps especially if they did not have a significant Labour presence. The variables used in this analysis, and a summary of the results, are given in Appendix Two.

The Labour Party was thus clearly associated with areas of working-class distress, and also with higher levels of spending on healthcare, but it is too simplistic to equate socialism with one single set of characteristics or policies. The ideology, administrative style and character of leading council personnel have all been identified as affecting the efficiency of some local parties over others in imposing their ideals on the council – whatever their party label.[65] The local political feeling also had an impact on the way in which Labour members expressed themselves, as will be seen with particular clarity in our case studies (Chapters four to seven). Trade unionism had a strong impact on the form the local Labour Party took in Gateshead and Barnsley. In Croydon, Labour politics had a more middle-class flavour. Local studies have supported the fact that local Labour parties might be quite different from each other in character and ideology, and this will be explored in greater detail in our own case studies as well. It is also important to note that at a national level, much progressive health legislation had been enacted by non-Labour governments: for example, the 1918 Maternity and Child Welfare Act, which was passed by David Lloyd George's Coalition government. The relationship between local and central politics is clearly another significant part of the explanation for how municipal politics developed in different towns, and one to which we now turn.

65 Powell, 'Did Politics Matter?', 368.

Central/Local Relations

The foregoing sections have hinted at the nature of relations between the localities and the central authority of the Ministry of Health in particular. It is clear that Ministry officials were keen to build up as complete a picture as possible of health care and decision making in the local authorities in the 1930s, but it also seems that the degree to which they could impose their own directives was limited. Ultimately they had little sanction if a local council had its own priorities: they could threaten to withhold agreement to loans or cut the central Exchequer grant, but in reality this was never enforced. It is worth dwelling on this relationship in a little more detail, as it explains a lot about the way that local policies were formed in this era of extreme localism, and will form an important part of the background to the case studies.[66]

The interwar period brought its own particular and growing tensions to the relationship between the Ministry and the individual County Boroughs because of the increasing duties placed on local authorities without any corresponding rise in independent income. The percentage of local authority income derived from central government grants rose from 30 per cent in 1920 to 44 per cent in 1938, giving the latter body (theoretically at least) greater influence in how it was spent.[67] This trend was strengthened in particular by the introduction of centrally apportioned block grants from 1929 – a system which also suggests that local problems were increasingly

66 This approach is worth stressing in the context of the 'Westminster narrative' which has been dominant in the historiography of the post-war era written by historians (although not political scientists). See R. Lowe and N. Rollings, 'Modernising Britain, 1957–64: A Classic Case of Centralisation and Fragmentation?' in R. A. W. Rhodes, ed., *Transforming British Government* i: *Changing Institutions* (London, 2000), 99.

67 M. Duprée, 'The Provision of Social Services' in M. Daunton, ed., *The Cambridge Urban History of Britain*, iii: *1840–1950* (Cambridge, 2000), 388. See also the discussion in Chapter One.

being reconceptualised as national ones even prior to 1939.[68] In fact, as has already been suggested, this shift was not really translated into firm action from the centre when it came to health.

This lack of assertiveness from the centre was not obvious in the way that the Ministry of Health was set up in 1919. George Newman, the Chief Medical Officer, heralded it as a major advance, and evidence that 'the national health is of supreme and vital importance' to both the individual and the nation as a whole.[69] Christopher Addison, the first Minister of Health, although apparently a 'dull' figure, nevertheless 'commanded much respect for his energy and enthusiasm, for his long connection with welfare policies ... and for his close political association with the Prime Minister.' He was a key figure in the post-war drive for the creation of a 'developmental state', as were Sir Robert Morant, who was to become the first Permanent Secretary to the Ministry, and George Newman, the Chief Medical Officer. Both Morant and Newman were seen as highly competent and dynamic administrators and among that 'most creative civil servants of the age.'[70]

Initially, then, the Ministry got off to a dynamic start, backing up its strong vision to improve the nation's health with a commitment to spend, as 'men's minds were turned towards projects for the development and extension' of clinics, dispensaries and other health services.[71] The Ministry's own publications gave the impression that this rosy picture continued throughout the interwar period, with the annual reports imparting a positive message, even during the years of retrenchment. For example, following the cuts of 1921, the Ministry described this time as an opportunity to survey the whole field of health services, so that when the economic

68 Lowe and Rollings 'Modernising Britain', 103. Ashford places this in a longer term context of, in welfare terms at least, the centre subordinating localities dating back at least to the Whig reforms of the first half of the nineteenth century: D. Ashford, *The Emergence of the Welfare States* (Oxford, 1986), 126, 117. J. Davis, 'Central Government and the Towns' in M. Daunton, ed., *The Cambridge Urban History of Britain*, iii: *1840–1950*, 279–81.

69 Annual Report of the Chief Medical Officer, 1919–20, Cmd. 978, xvii, p. 7.

70 K. O. Morgan, *Consensus and Disunity: The Lloyd George Coalition Government, 1918–22* (Oxford, 1986), 82, 84.

71 Second Annual Report of the Ministry of Health, 1920–21, Cmd. 1446, xiii, p. 1.

circumstances permitted fresh progress to be made, policies would be based upon 'a mature and deliberate plan.'[72] Its optimistic outlook was further underpinned by the ongoing improvement in the nation's health. The 1937 Annual Report cited the improvement in housing, the better 'personal habits' of individuals, and the expansion of personal services supporting the health of the population which 'between them embrace the seven ages of man, from cradle to grave.'[73] In consequence of these improvements, it claimed, adults and, especially children, now enjoyed 'a healthier and fuller life than at any time since the Industrial Revolution.'[74]

But there was a more problematic reality behind the almost relentless optimism propagated by the Chief Medical Officers of Health through their Annual Reports. Welshman has noted the serious doubts raised by several high-profile contemporaries, including Sir Arthur Newsholme, the ex-Chief Medical Officer of the Local Government Board (the body replaced by the Ministry of Health).[75] None of this was helped by the spending cuts of the early 1920s – the 'Geddes Axe' – which not only had an impact on services but also led to the cut of a third of civil servants employed in the Ministry.[76] This meant that not only was its ability to expand services drastically curtailed, but also that its capacity to enforce existing policies was reduced. One senior official stated that while cuts had affected all central departments, 'I doubt whether it has been felt in any Department to the same degree as in the Ministry of Health.'[77] In such circumstances, it is perhaps understandable that local authorities could hold out against the centre, if determined to pursue their own agenda.

72 Ibid, 1.

73 While most indicators of health – infant mortality rates, deaths from infectious diseases, life expectancy – showed an improvement over the period, maternal mortality was the major exception. For a discussion of this point see C. Webster, 'Healthy or Hungry Thirties?' *History Workshop Journal*, 8 (1982), also his 'Health, Welfare and the Unemployed During the Depression', *Past and Present*, 109 (1985).

74 Eighteenth Annual Report of the Ministry of Health, 1936–1937: Cmd.5516, p. x, viii.

75 Quoted in Welshman, *Municipal Medicine*, 253.

76 J. E. Pater, *The Making of the National Health Service* (London, 1981), 10.

77 I. G. Gibbons, 'The Ministry of Health' *Journal of Public Administration*, 4:3 (1926), 259.

The Ministry was further weighed down by the wide nature of its remit. Although named the 'Ministry of Health', it actually had responsibilities over anything related to local government and its interaction with the central state – a hangover from the transfer of responsibilities from the old Local Government Board.[78] Morant, the first Permanent Secretary, could have been a dynamic force towards unification and progress, but as S. Stacey has argued, his unexpected death in 1921, coupled with Addison's political demise and the more general context of renewed administrative and fiscal conservatism, dealt a fatal blow to plans for a dynamic and forward-looking Ministry.[79] Arthur Robinson, Morant's successor, was a generalist of the old school and remained in post until 1940. In short, as Webster has asserted, from its early promise, the Ministry of Health became, by the mid-1920s, a 'career backwater staffed by second-rate minds suitable to act only as instruments of regulation.'[80] This, again, led to a weakening of central direction, and room for local independence, as Welshman has shown effectively for Leicester.[81] The Victorian system of negotiation, rather than rule by decree, remained.[82]

The health surveys of the 1930s reflect the Ministry's position as advisor rather than master; but this seems to have been a matter of choice. Newman himself noted in 1919, for example, that relationships with local

78 For some observers, even at the point of creation the Ministry was the 'outcome of a matrimonial union consummated in 1919 between the old aristocratic Local Government Board and the new plutocratic Insurance Commission, with Dr Addison presiding over the ceremony and Sir Robert Morant acting as best man.': Gibbons, 'The Ministry of Health', 243. See also S. R. Stacey, 'The Ministry of Health, 1919–29: Ideas and Practice in a Government Department', DPhil thesis, University of Oxford, 1984, 1.

79 Stacey 'The Ministry of Health', 77.

80 Webster 'Conflict and Consensus', 142–7.

81 Welshman *Municipal Medicine*, 252.

82 Davis, 'Central Government and the Towns', 263. See also M. Beloff, 'The Whitehall Factor: The Role of the Higher Civil Service 1919–39', in G. Peele and C. Cook, eds, *The Politics of Reappraisal, 1918–39* (London, 1975); R. Davidson and R. Lowe, 'Bureaucracy and Innovation in British Welfare Policy 1890–1945' in W. J. Mommsen, ed., *The Emergence of the Welfare State in Britain and Germany, 1850–1950* (London, 1981).

authorities were 'built on the basis of assent and consent rather than on compulsion.'[83] Instead, the Ministry promoted information sharing, for example via the publication of annual league tables of costs relating to TB care, which it hoped would prompt local authorities to compare the value of their services to other similar administrative units.[84] This seems to have been effective insofar as borough councils did frequently cite how the costs of their services measured up to others'.[85] However, as we have seen, wide variation remained, suggesting that the Ministry was not able (or inclined) to push a levelling agenda. The Annual Reports were another means of promoting information exchange, for example to suggest greater co-operation between individual councils and voluntary hospitals and organisations. Indeed, one of the strongest themes to emerge from the 1930s surveys was the desire to consider health services in the round; not merely to push the expansion of the municipal sector. As the Ministry Annual Report of 1933 pointed out, local authorities did not as yet realise 'how many and varied are the services which they might well accept from voluntary agencies in the matter of organisation, in detail of administration and in general support.'[86]

Despite these prompts to further action, the fact remained that the Ministry had very little real power during this period. The majority of health legislation passed in the interwar years was permissive rather than compulsory, and as a result much actual policy decision making, as well as implementation, was left to the discretion of the localities. This led to considerable frustration among Ministry officials, who felt that the sorts of internal squabbling cited in the section on hospital appropriation above were a distraction from the bigger picture of healthcare. Officials com-

83 Supplement Containing the Report of the Medical Department for 1918–19 (as part of Local Government Board 48th Annual Report) 1919, Cmd. 462, vi.

84 These tables can be found in TNA MH96/1114–1116, Welsh National Memorial Association, comparative TB institution costs, 1922–39.

85 See Chapter Five, for an example of Eastbourne comparing its levels of expenditure to the other coastal resort towns of Hastings and Bournemouth.

86 On the State of the Public Health. Annual Report of the Chief Medical Officer (London, 1933), p. 89.

plained of the 'antagonism arising either as a result of vested interests or mistaken sense of so called civic pride', particularly when urging smaller authorities to enter into common schemes to share facilities.[87] On the other side, however, some boroughs felt that the Ministry was overly concerned with the minutiae of daily service provision. Its officers engaged in lengthy correspondence with Newport, for example, over whether or not it was appropriate for the MOH to also act as police surgeon,[88] and with West Hartlepool on the question of the positioning of the door of its VD clinic.[89] The Ministry's role and stated aims were thus contradictory; at once in favour of local independence, and overly engaged with sometimes petty details. This certainly hampered its ability to promote a uniform approach to the development of health services in this period. Nonetheless, low-level monitoring and guidance were in many cases effective, at least where the local authority was amenable to it. Our case studies will indicate that in boroughs with more entrenched attitudes the Ministry rapidly ran out of options.

A similar 'guiding' approach was taken by the Welsh Board of Health, which could produce antagonism locally from those who resented instruction from the centre, albeit at a devolved level. For example, in its correspondence on Newport County Borough, the representative suggested that further enquiries should be 'cut down to the minimum and Newport left to work out their own salvation.'[90] In Wales, however the situation was complicated by the existence of another Welsh-wide healthcare body, the

87 TNA MH96/1064, Anti-TB Inquiry Report. Brief Prepared by the Welsh Board of Health for the Minister 20 March 1939. Although this was flagged up in relation to smaller sanitary authorities it is quite clear that the same problems also existed between larger authorities. Such a case was the prolonged development of the Poole Joint Sanatorium, which was finally established on the outskirts of Middlesbrough in the late 1930s to serve the TB patients of six County Boroughs in the north-east.

88 TNA MH96/387, Survey Report, Newport.

89 TNA, MH66/991 and MH66/995, Survey Correspondence and Resurvey Correspondence, West Hartlepool.

90 TNA MH96/388, Survey Correspondence, Newport, minute, Dr Low, 9 August 1933. It should be added that this was because the borough seemed likely to make improvements under its own initiative.

King Edward VII Welsh National Memorial Association. This was a voluntary body (although the local authorities were the major contributors to its funds) which from 1921 took on the provision of all services except aftercare for TB cases in Welsh County Boroughs and County Councils.[91] This meant that, unlike in England, local authorities did not have full decision making powers over the whole range of health services, but instead had to work with another provider. It is clear that some of the Welsh authorities found this difficult. One MOH, for example, complained in the early 1920s that medical work in his borough was divided between his own department, the School Medical Service and the Welsh National Memorial Association. This led to 'much overlapping of efforts in many directions, a large amount of unnecessary clerical work ... ignorance on the part of one dept in reference to the work of others, and much unnecessary work in the visitation of homes by different officials.'[92] Certainly the Welsh Board of Health was criticised by contemporaries for its ineffectual nature. After carrying out a TB Inquiry in 1939 Clement Davies, Liberal National MP for Montgomeryshire, described it as a 'useless moribund organisation', and as a 'National Waste Paper Basket' where reports of medical officers and sanitary inspectors were discarded.[93]

It is clear that despite its promising start and rhetoric of action and success, the Ministry of Health – and also the Welsh Board of Health – were extremely limited in the extent to which they could impose direc-

91 TNA MH96/1099, Newport County Borough Council: Treatment of Tuberculosis Scheme 1920–1930, Circular 190 (Wales), Ministry of Health & Welsh Board of Health, 25 May 1921. For a more general exploration of the role the Welsh National Memorial Association took in TB provision in Wales, see L. Bryder, 'The King Edward VII Welsh National Memorial Association and its Policy Towards Tuberculosis, 1910–48', *Welsh History Review*, 13:2(1986).

92 TNA MH96/1099, Newport County Borough Council: Treatment of Tuberculosis Scheme 1920–1930, 'Coordination of Public Health Services at Newport', Report by the MOH, Dr J. Howard Jones.

93 TNA MH55/1198, Anti-tuberculosis committee for Wales: observation on Reports; *Western Mail, The Times*, 3 April 1939, quoted in L. Bryder 'The King Edward VII Welsh National Memorial Association', 210. 'Clement Davies', *Dictionary of National Biography*, [online] <http://www.oxforddnb.com/> accessed 16 April 2010.

tion on local authorities where they were not willing to listen. Yet at the same time the local authorities themselves seem, in certain circumstances, to have appreciated the role taken by the Ministry of Health, which was able to negotiate and use its status to push local authority cooperation. A representative of South Shields County Borough, for example, stated in the context of negotiations over a joint TB sanatorium in the north-east, that 'the probability of the local authorities concerned agreeing to attend such a conference *is much greater if the conference is called by the Ministry rather than by my council*' [emphasis added].[94] And this was not an isolated example. In West Hartlepool the suggestion of increased cooperation between council health services and local voluntary hospitals led a representative to argue that if the recommendation came from West Hartlepool Corporation then it 'would be resented, and would be rejected at once. But, if it came from the Ministry, he felt sure that it would be considered.'[95] Clearly then, the Ministry was valued at some level, giving weight and prestige to certain proposals and perhaps able to generate a degree of momentum that a single authority alone would find hard. In this sense the Ministry of Health did succeed in performing one of the roles envisaged for it by its creators. However, it is also clear that the simple dichotomy between 'the council' and 'the centre' needs a more sophisticated and careful reading, as well as a deeper understanding of how the agency of councils was expressed in its relationship with the centre. This is one of the purposes of our case studies, which we now move on to contextualise.

94 TNA MH67/133, Proposed Joint Sanatorium: Conference of Local Authorities: Appendices: Survey of Resources of Area, 1930–1931, South Shields to Ministry of Health, 15 December 1930.

95 TNA MH66/993, Resurvey Report West Hartlepool, 23.

The Selection of Four Case Studies

The analysis based on aggregate expenditure and national-level data has highlighted a number of features and explanations for spending on municipal health services. It has also flagged up a wide array of factors which were very significant in shaping local decisions, but which are not readily quantifiable in the sense of lending themselves to statistical testing. This is where case studies which use a much wider and more detailed array of sources come into their own, particularly when contextualised in the larger-scale national-level data. In this case, we have been able to use the national data to select case studies which spotlight some of the wider emerging themes.

There were two central criteria for selecting case studies. The first was population size: for practical reasons, an upper limit of 100,000 inhabitants at the start of the interwar period was set. It would simply not have been possible to carry out four contrasting studies in the time available if each had the data and complexity of a large borough like Manchester or Birmingham, with their multiple institutions, and sub-urban level patterns of local health care provision. The second, and more hypothesis-driven factor, was the desire to include boroughs which between them filled all four areas in a quadrant: rich, poor, low Labour, high Labour. This would allow us to unpick further the reality of local provision, within a context of that difficult-to-explain conundrum of Labour/high needs/high expenditure which was outlined above.

The case studies were thus selected by creating yearly scatter plots depicting rateable value and Labour representation for all boroughs in the specified population bracket.[96] The plots for each year were compared, and four boroughs were selected on the basis of how well they fitted our quadrant characteristics. The selection of the case studies was thus based on statistical characteristics, and not available sources. While our case studies fit our aims, there were undoubtedly others which could have served

96 We used z-scores in these plots, which show how each borough performed relative to the mean for the sample.

as well; however, since it is clear that each borough has its own distinctive characteristics, there is in a sense, no 'wrong' choice. In each case, a backup borough was identified in case the first choices turned out not to have rich enough sources, but in the event they were not needed. Figure 3.6 sets out how the final four case studies fit into our quadrant framework.

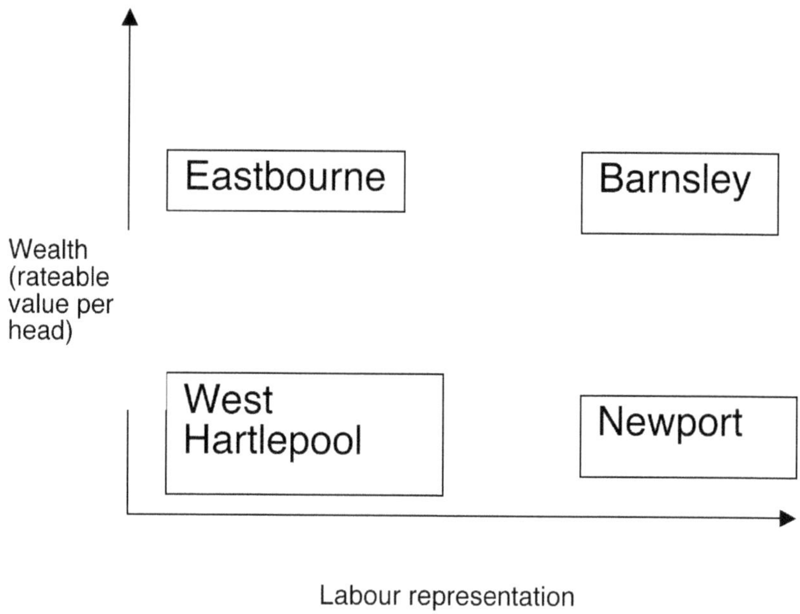

Figure 3.6 The Selection of Four Case-Study Boroughs
Source: Local Government Financial Statistics; The *Times* annual election reports, 1922/3–1936/7

Eastbourne – a resort town on the south coast – was consistently a rich borough with low Labour representation across the period. It also spent well above the average on health services, particularly at the start of the period (indeed, it was a significant outlier on all of the factors used for selection). Its status as a seaside resort also introduced the question of whether it had particular socio-economic characteristics which would both have directed health policy, and dictated its needs. Barnsley, in the

West Riding of Yorkshire, was also a high spending borough, but it was a town with strong Labour associations, and a much poorer socio-economic profile than Eastbourne in terms of rateable values. Its high expenditure levels are thus likely to be the result of quite a different set of priorities and decisions. It was the only one of the four case studies to appropriate a hospital. Newport, in Monmouthshire (Wales) was also a town with a high proportion of Labour councillors (around 40 per cent of seats, and a majority in three years of the period), but it did not spend at a very high level on health services despite relatively buoyant rateable values. However, its expenditure did rise over the second half of the period. Its Welsh location was a further factor in its selection from the possible case studies in this quadrant, because of the distinctively different provision for TB services there. Finally, West Hartlepool, in the North-East, was neither a high spending, nor particularly Labour-influenced borough, and had relatively poor indicators of wealth. According to our quadrant, it had neither of the spurs to high expenditure.

Further details on the key selection characteristics of the four towns are set out in Figure 3a–e. Figure 3a presents population levels, which were relatively stable in all four towns, although with some decline in Newport in the later part of the period. Figure 3b shows just how much of an outlier Eastbourne was in terms of wealth (rateable values), especially after the 1929 Local Government Act, while West Hartlepool and Barnsley had little to distinguish them in terms of poor resources. Newport almost exactly reflected the County Borough average. Figure 3c makes the same point for Labour representation on the councils, although some of the more marked dips and troughs (most notably the early jump in West Hartlepool) may be the result of misreporting – as is commented on in greater detail in the chapter on that town. Together, the graphs in Figure 3 indicate the range of experience in terms of the background characteristics which governed the selection of the case studies. Figure 3d illustrates the range in levels of expenditure across the case studies, and also that there were some shifts in the trends over the period. Newport, for example, became an above average spender after 1930, while Barnsley's outlay shot up in 1936 (the result of the appropriation of its transferred institution). West Hartlepool and Eastbourne were more constant in their spending levels across the period, at low and high levels, respectively. Finally, Figure 3e gives us our first suggestion of how complex the relationship between politics, wealth and outlay was. In terms of the rate actually set in the pound, the residents of rich, high spending Eastbourne had little demanded of them, while Barnsley set the rate burden of its residents much higher. Newport increased the level of rate set over the period, while West Hartlepool made cuts. These patterns suggest very different experiences for ratepayers and different priorities for council members. Finally, Table 3.1 presents data on expenditure on different health services in the four case-study towns, with a measure of how these relate to the mean for the national dataset (the z-score), and also a measure of how they changed over the period. This illustrates the variability of experience within each borough, and provides some background for the detailed examination which follows. We have not attempted to be exhaustive in our analysis of local healthcare provision in our case studies. Instead, we have expanded on the most influential factors setting up decision making and expenditure in each case. Other areas of health care provision were provided for and debated locally, but as a study in identifying the workings of local government, we hope we need make no apology for this focus.

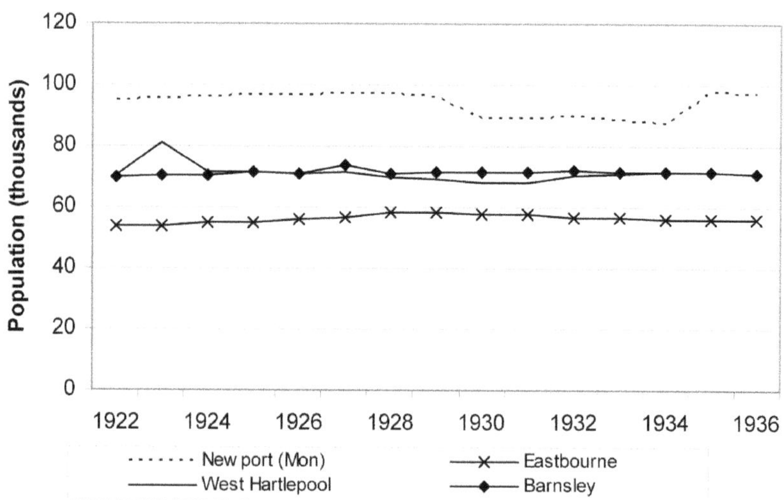

Figure 3.7a Population of Four Case-Study Boroughs, 1922–36
Source: Local Government Financial Statistics

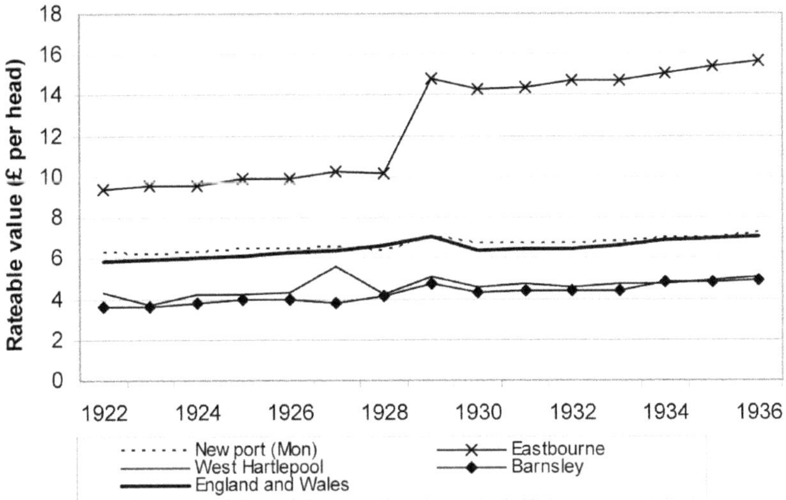

Figure 3.7b Rateable Value per Head in Four Case-Study Boroughs, 1922–36
Source: as above

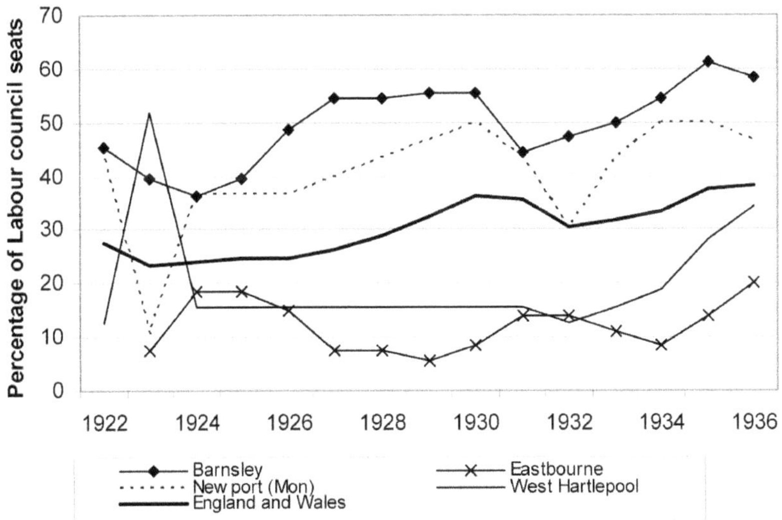

Figure 3.7c Percentage of Council Seats Held by Labour in Four Case-Study Boroughs, 1922–36
Source: The *Times* municipal election reports

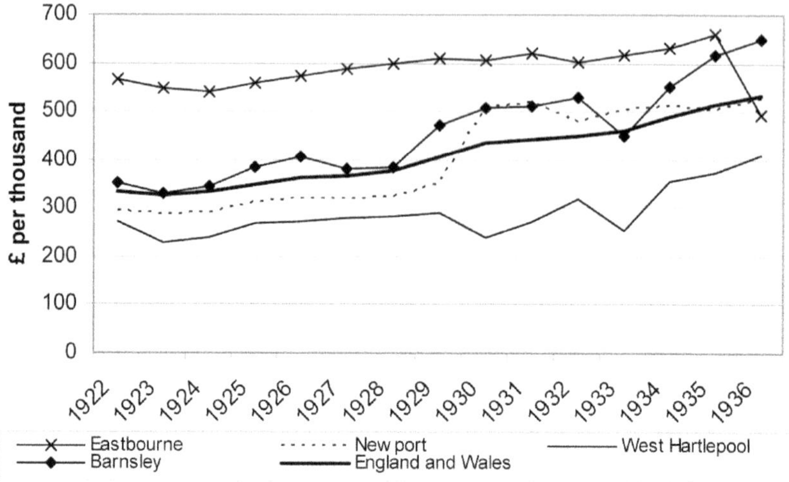

Figure 3.7d Expenditure per Thousand on Personal Health Services in Four Case-Study Boroughs, 1922–36
Source: as above

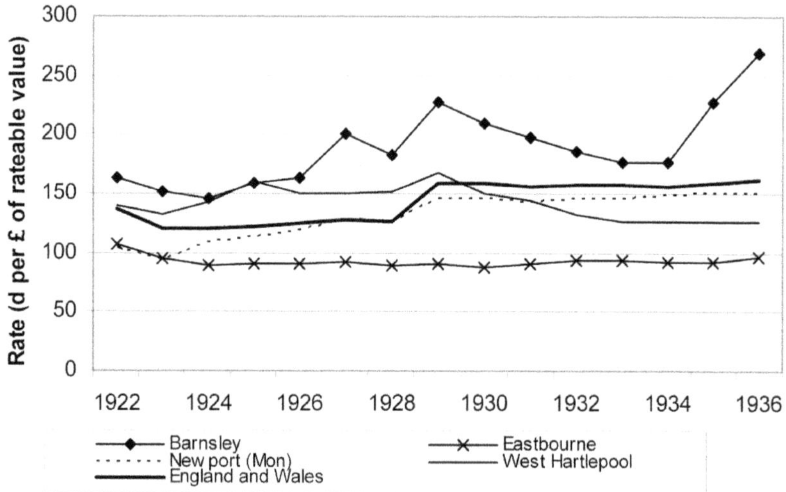

Figure 3.7e Amount of Rate Levied in the Pound in Four Case-Study Boroughs, 1922–36
Source: Local Government Financial Statistics

	1922 expenditure	1922 z-score	1936 expenditure	1936 z-score	change from 1922 to 1936
Mental hospitals					
Barnsley	13.5	-0.837	20.6	-0.486	7.0
Eastbourne	201.4	3.643	76.0	0.696	-125.4
Newport	71.5	0.544	51.1	0.164	-20.4
West Hartlepool	93.4	1.066	9.0	-0.732	-84.4
Mental deficiency					
Barnsley	12.3	-0.134	50.3	-0.509	37.9
Eastbourne	15.3	0.149	57.9	-0.347	42.5
Newport	5.4	-0.786	38.2	-0.770	32.8
West Hartlepool	6.3	-0.699	55.9	-0.389	49.6
TB					
Barnsley	70.9	-0.137	113.2	0.011	42.3
Eastbourne	110.6	0.826	94.5	-0.467	-16.1
Newport	23.0	-1.300	131.8	0.485	108.8
West Hartlepool	71.8	-0.115	62.2	-1.294	-9.6
MCW					
Barnsley	73.0	1.127	144.6	1.194	71.7
Eastbourne	97.1	2.202	122.1	0.597	25.0
Newport	40.0	-0.345	107.9	0.221	67.9
West Hartlepool	34.4	-0.596	79.3	-0.536	45.0
Infectious disease					
Barnsley	126.3	1.305	212.0	3.468	85.8
Eastbourne	99.8	0.563	90.6	-0.116	-9.2
Newport	78.7	-0.026	98.1	0.105	19.4
West Hartlepool	13.9	-1.837	97.0	0.075	83.1

	1922 expenditure	1922 z-score	1936 expenditure	1936 z-score	change from 1922 to 1936
Total health					
Barnsley	351.2	0.167	890.5	0.935	539.3
Eastbourne	566.7	2.289	493.1	-0.780	-73.6
Newport	292.8	-0.407	524.7	-0.643	231.9
West Hartlepool	272.9	-0.603	408.5	-1.145	135.6

Table 3.1 Expenditure per Thousand on Major Municipal Health Services in Four Case-Study Boroughs, 1922 and 1936
Source: Local Government Financial Statistics

CHAPTER FOUR

Barnsley*

Barnsley fulfils all of the most stereotyped characteristics of a County Borough town in the interwar period: poor, northern, depressed, dependent on one industry, and providing an unhealthy environment for its residents. Lying in the heart of the South Yorkshire coalfield, it was hard hit by the decline in the mining industry after World War One. It was also a very political place, with strong Labour representation, and an active trade union and co-operative workers' movement. Yet despite its relative poverty – and perhaps because of its political colour – it spent above the average County Borough rate per head on health services. This chapter will try to unpick the inter-relations between these different factors, focusing on the strength and nature of the local Labour Party, the high levels of socio-economic and medical need in the town, and the significance of local traditions and individuals in shaping municipal decisions on healthcare.

The socio-economic and environmental position of the town certainly meant that Barnsley had great need of a good health service. The Ministry of Health inspector who visited the town in 1932 and 1933 painted an unpromising picture:

> In general appearance Barnsley is ... one of the most sordid and depressing towns in England. There are few buildings or streets ... its open spaces are said to consist mostly of waste ground on which buildings cannot be erected owing to the danger of mining subsidence ... [The] main feature of the town is an enormous slag heap ... [which] is in a continual state of spontaneous combustion and emits the most nauseating sulphurous fumes.[1]

* The authors would like to thank Cllr Michael Stokes, Barnsley MBC, for his help, time and assistance in accessing the records of Barnsley Labour Party and Trades Council (with which it merged in 1919).

1 TNA MH66/1066, Survey Report, Barnsley, 1–2. The inspector, Dr Wilkinson, visited the town between 12–16 December 1932 and 23–27 January 1933.

On top of this came the occupational instability – not to say health risks – attendant on the coal mining industry, which employed 44 per cent of the male population in 1931.[2] This sector had suffered a drop in productivity when wartime demand ended, and this was exacerbated by Germany's re-entry into the market after the Dawes Plan of 1925. Jobs and pay were insecure, and industrial unrest culminated in the 1926 General Strike, when a quarter of the population was in receipt of poor relief. The sector had barely recovered before the onset of the depression.[3] In December 1932 one fifth of the population was receiving either dole or public assistance, with 3386 on Outdoor Relief, and about another four thousand on Transitional Benefit.[4]

These social, economic and health problems were exacerbated by the poor state of the houses inhabited by the working classes. George Orwell described the problems in Barnsley in *The Road to Wigan Pier*, based on a visit made in the spring of 1936. It is significant for our purposes that he particularly cites the powerlessness – or perhaps disinterest – of the council in making improvements. He wrote of one home:

> Walls very bad – wall of back room cracked right through. Window frames coming to pieces and have to be stuffed with wood. Rain comes through in several places. Sewer runs under house and stinks in summer but Corporation 'says they can't do nowt.' Six people in house, two adults and four children, the eldest aged fifteen. Youngest but one attending hospital – tuberculosis suspected. House infested by bugs. Rent 5s.3d, including rates.[5]

The Ministry of Health inspector also noted the severe overcrowding of working-class homes (although he excepted the council built accommodation), particularly in the central ward which was said to be most densely

2 S. Davies and B. Morley, *County Borough Elections in England and Wales, 1919–1938*, i: *Barnsley–Bournemouth* (Aldershot, 1999), Appendix nine.

3 Eighth Annual Report of the Ministry of Health, 1926–7, Cmd. 2938, ix, pp. 127–8.

4 TNA MH66/1066, Survey Report, Barnsley, 4.

5 George Orwell *The Road to Wigan Pier* (New Edn, London, 1989), 49–50.

populated place in the West Riding.[6] This is reflected also in the rapid population growth over our period: from 53,661 inhabitants in 1921, to 71,522 in 1931.[7] Barnsley's population was a young one: birth rates were high, as were maternal and infant mortality rates, all again pointing to large families with many children, and poor indicators of both environmental and personal health.

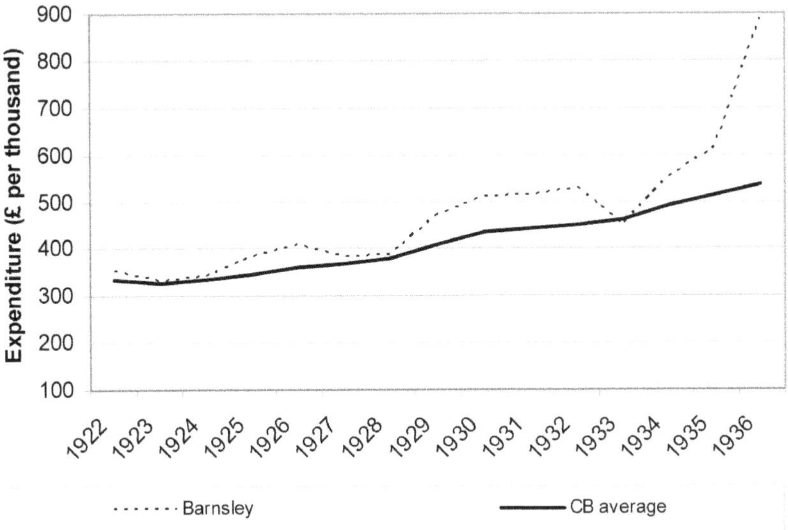

Figure 4.1 Expenditure per Thousand on Health, Barnsley County Borough, 1922/3–36/7
Source: Local Government Financial statistics, 1922/23–36/7

Barnsley did, however, respond to these poor conditions with above average levels of investment in personal health services. We will see that this was in marked contrast with other poorly off boroughs like West Hartlepool. As Figure 4.1 indicates, the borough consistently spent at least the national average per thousand of its population on the personal health services, and

6 TNA MH66/1066, Survey Report, Barnsley, 4–5.
7 Population figures are from the 1921 and 1931 Censuses for England and Wales.

frequently above. This was especially true in the years following the 1929 Local Government Act, while the large spike in 1935 was the result of the appropriation of its transferred institution. At this stage per capita spending even overtook Eastbourne – our 'rich, high spending' case study, which was then experiencing a sharp downturn (see Chapter Five).

The above-average levels of expenditure on health are even more noteworthy when we consider that Barnsley's property base had the lowest rateable value of all of our case studies: a third below the national average. At the same time, the council also levied the highest rates in the pound of all four towns for the whole period: 16 shillings compared with a national average of 12 shillings (see Figures 3.7b and e, Chapter Three). Whereas rich Eastbourne did not need to tax its residents highly in order to maintain a good income from rates, Barnsley had to ask much more of taxpayers. That it did so reflects an inclination to respond to high levels of need: other poorly off boroughs, like West Hartlepool, would not risk their residents' wrath by raising rates.

This commitment to investment in ameliorative services is one associated with left-wing politics, and Barnsley's council did have a large number of Labour councillors from the start of the period (see Figure 4.2). Indeed, Barnsley has maintained its reputation as a Labour stronghold well into the twenty-first century. The party never held less than 38 per cent of council seats during the interwar years (the national average was closer to 25 per cent until the late 1920s), although it only had an outright majority between November 1927 and November 1930, and from 1933 onwards. In 1926–7 and 1932–3 there were hung councils, which gave Labour a significant voice, but no absolute mandate to lead. From 1930 to 1932 the Independents (as the local alliance of conservatives styled themselves) were in control. We will see that politics did play a significant part in the spending decisions of this council, and that Labour representatives particularly prioritised certain needs-based health services, as our theoretical framework would predict.

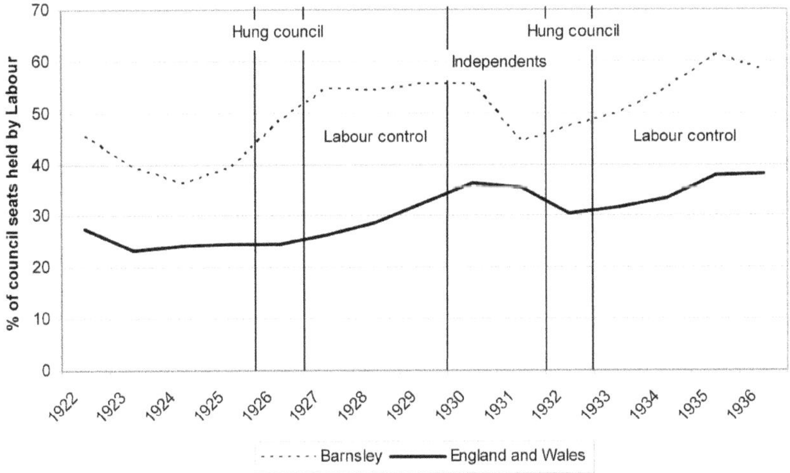

Figure 4.2 Percentage of Labour Seats on Barnsley Council, 1922–36
Source: *The Times* municipal election returns, 1922–36.
Note: these dates show the calendar year, rather than the financial year – therefore 1930 represents the financial year of 1929–30.

The Labour Party and Municipal Spending in Barnsley

Labour not only had a strong presence in Barnsley; it was also a combative and well organised political grouping, with a strong party line on certain issues. This included a commitment to many of the health services which benefited the working classes in particular, such as MCW. It was noted in previous chapters that this is the relationship found in other studies, but it was not necessarily a given in interwar municipal politics; local Labour parties were not all of a piece, and Barnsley's was much better organised and unified than its equivalents in either Newport or West Hartlepool. Although party colour cannot explain all of the decisions made in Barnsley, the local Labour Party gave consistently the strongest impetus and direction to action in this town.

The reason for the assertive and focussed action of Barnsley's Labour Party seems to have been its strong leadership. Work on Barnsley's leading Labour figures has tended to be dominated by hagiography, however it does appear that certain individuals – Andrew Wright, Edward Sheerien, Joseph Jones and the miners' leader Herbert Smith – were key in maintaining order and setting the agenda.[8] Sheerien is a particularly significant figure for our current study, as he was also the Chair of the Health Committee (as well as chairing several other committees, including finance – often the key committee in local government at this time – and education) and was the Secretary of the local party until 1954.[9] He also took a strong socialist stance on healthcare and its primary functions:

> Sheerien had a saying 'consider what the people need, not what they want.' He saw the slums, he saw Barnsley top of the infant mortality league, and he thought out a post-war plan to deal with the problems. It was a black and white plan – no compromise. 'He had vision, but was not imaginative', was the comment of a protégé of his. Thus he carried out the plan the only way he knew. He created a machine, and forced the town to have what it needed. He said 'We have to have power for a long time.'[10]

This statement gives a clear flavour of Labour politics under Sheerien's direction: namely, it was committed to retaining power so that it could push through a unified plan which would address the most pressing social needs of the borough. It is also clear that this plan would be followed in the face of objections. Sheerien's mode of action was 'autocratic', as one party member remembered: 'If Sheerien's hand went up, all went up, if they

8 See in particular, J. Watts and D. Nannestad, *The First Fifty Years – Half a Century of Labour Rule in Barnsley* (Barnsley, 1983). Watts is the grand-daughter of Edward Sheerien. A slightly more critical approach can be found in T. Lindley, 'The Party Machine: A Study of Barnsley Labour Party and its Leaders, 1918–1945', dissertation for the Social Studies Diploma, Ruskin College, 1978. Lindley describes the roles of these principal men as: 'Jones the front man, Sheerien the organiser and Wright the fixer' (58).

9 Watts and Nannestad, *The First Fifty Years*, 8.

10 Lindley, 'The Party Machine', 18. Sheerien was elected to the council in 1923, from a background on the Trades Council, where he was a delegate and then secretary for the Shop Assistants' Union.

didn't he wouldn't forget.' Sheerien, Jones and Wright 'were not averse to removing a Chairman from his chair or a member from a Committee if they transgressed. Even the great Herbert Smith had the whip withdrawn on at least one occasion'.[11]

The local Labour Party thus had a clear programme of political demands, and it also sustained separate Housing and Health Committees, which further indicates some of its main priorities.[12] Its influence was boosted by the fact that municipal politics in Barnsley generally were unstable and adversarial. Labour manipulated this to its advantage whenever it could, for example reneging on promises in order to manipulate the aldermanic system and mayoralty and thus gain influence, and boycotting the Public Assistance Committee in years when they were not given equal representation on it (even though they were at that stage in the minority on the council).[13] Whenever Labour was in the majority, even if it was only by one councillor, its representatives pressed for reform. This supports Powell's assessment of the importance of the *style* of Labour administration in shaping local politics, especially when compared with our other Labour-influenced case study, Newport.[14] By 1937 Labour representatives held all Committee chairmanships on the council, and had ended the pact under which the position of Mayor alternated between parties: 'Socialists do not make pacts with non-socialists' said Sheerien, and the new policy was brought in despite complaints from the opposition. In fact, the opposition soon formed itself into the Citizens'

11 Labour Party informant quoted in Lindley, 'The Party Machine', 35, 55.

12 BALS A/1963/G/1, Barnsley Trades Union Council and Labour Party Minute Book 1916–20. In the majority of boroughs housing was subsumed within the Health Committee.

13 For example, in 1938 on the death of two councillors, Herbert Smith and John Potts, Labour's majority was down to two. The Party decided that rather than risk losing control they would elect a non-councillor to the aldermanic vacancy. This led to the appointment of the first Labour woman to sit on the council, Mrs Ann Elizabeth Marsh, who had been an early member of the Independent Labour Party, was active in the Trade Union Movement and was chair of the local Women's Section.

14 M. Powell, 'Did Politics Matter? Municipal Public Health Expenditure in the 1930s', *Urban History*, 22:3 (1995).

Party to provide a united anti-Labour front, indicating something of the perception of Labour among those who did not support it.[15]

However, it is not enough simply to think about the influence of individuals, albeit powerful ones, on Barnsley's Labour Party: we need to consider the labour movement in its broader sense. Thus the party also received direction from the Trades Council, which underpinned the whip system in place for Labour councillors from 1930, while individual trade unions and the cooperative movement were also very significant.[16] In fact it is impossible to underestimate the influence of the miners' associations in Barnsley and in the Labour Party during this period. The YMA and then the National Union of Mineworkers dominated the Parliamentary Labour Party in the area, and were key forces in municipal politics well into the mid-1980s. The YMA was a paternalistic union which provided its own leisure facilities and housing, and it also expected its Labour representatives on the council to push its agenda on a range of non-workplace issues including housing, welfare and health.[17] The co-operative movement was a further influence on the local Labour Party: it subsidised a number of strikes, ran credit schemes and also funded the party directly.[18] This gave Labour a very different ethos from its counterpart councillors in Newport.

Barnsley's Labour Party was thus influential, combative and well organised, and it had significant backing (and direction) from the various trades unions and co-operatives in the town. Together these forces had a

15 Watts and Nannestad, *The First Fifty Years*, 15. Similarly, non-Labour councillors in West Hartlepool were explicitly banding together as 'Moderates' by 1936 in an attempt to counter the growth of Labour as a political force.

16 Lindley, 'The Party Machine', 24.

17 Interview with Cllr Michael Stokes, Barnsley Metropolitan Borough Council, 11 August 2004 and 21 August 2004. An example is the way that the YMA actively sought representation on the board of the voluntary hospital, with all local Trade Union branches subsequently paying in a regular levy. BALSA/1963/G/1, Barnsley Trades Union Council and Labour Party Minute Book 1916–20, meetings of February 25 1920 and 24 November 1920.

18 The co-operative movement was one of the strong-holds of the Catholic section of the Labour Party (which was significant in Barnsley), and where Sheerien found the base of his support.

considerable impact on some of the municipal health services in particular, and tended to prompt high levels of investment whenever the party was in power. It is no coincidence that the periods of Labour majority on the council witnessed significant rises in spending on the MCW schemes, pay rises for nursing and health visitor staff, and the appropriation of Gawber Road PAI. Outside the field of health it saw a rapid increase in the building of housing, the implementation of a forty-hour week for council employees, attempts to raise the school leaving age to fourteen and a half, and to establish a municipal bank.[19] In the remainder of this section we will focus on the MCW services to illustrate the interplay between Labour's objectives and its implementation of health policies in particular.

MCW services can be regarded as instrumental in raising the bar for disadvantaged families, and so it is not surprising to see that an active Labour Party made them a priority. It is worth noting again, however, that this is not the only explanation for spending levels on any particular service, as was demonstrated in the national level data. Neither is it necessarily an indicator of quality *per se*. Barnsley spent well above the County Borough average on MCW services *throughout* the period, but there was a particular peak in spending in 1926 and generally sustained growth from 1932, which were both periods of Labour ascendancy. And yet despite generous investment, the services attracted unfavourable notice from Ministry of Health visitors: Dame Janet Campbell visited the town in 1931 and recorded that 'the Maternity and Child Welfare scheme as a whole needs a great deal of improvement before it can be looked upon satisfactorily.'[20]

19 Lindley, 'The Party Machine', 49–50.

20 TNA MH66/420, Survey Report, Barnsley, Appendices, Appendix S. Health Visitor visits to under-ones were unexceptional in number, up until 1933 the infant welfare centres were unattractive and of poor quality, and it took until 1934 before the presentation of new babies at an infant welfare clinic reached 73 per cent. Antenatal attendances remained below the County Borough average until 1936, and it was not until 1937 that 70 per cent, of expectant mothers attended the clinics. V. Cutts, 'Health During the Inter-War Period in the Mining Town of Barnsley', dissertation, Leeds University, 1981 [degree unspecified], 22–3.

One of the reasons for the mismatch between the amount of money spent on the entire service and its indifferent quality was the fact that much of the budget went disproportionately into providing free and subsidised milk to infants and expectant mothers. This was a scheme which had been prioritised before Labour took control of the council, but the Party was instrumental in maintaining it in the face of Ministry of Health opposition towards the end of our period. Between a fifth and a quarter of the total spent on MCW services in this borough went on the milk scheme. In 1933 this exceeded the equivalent in Eastbourne by a factor of ten, and in West Hartlepool by a factor of twenty five. Unlike other parts of the MCW budget like rent and salaries, which were largely fixed, milk provision was responsive to local economic conditions. As a result it was peculiarly susceptible to political decision making.

The commitment to free and subsidised milk was borne out of a desire to feed all children who needed it, regardless of cost. This led to several clashes with the Ministry of Health, who felt that the scheme was too generous, especially after the Geddes axe fell in 1922. Despite attempts to reduce Ministry contributions Barnsley stuck to its position and consequently continued to receive the higher level of subsidy throughout the early 1920s.[21] When the Ministry refused to award a supplementary grant to cover increased costs in 1926 (the year of the General Strike) the Council voted to bear the extra sum from the rates, again indicating its commitment to the benefits of this particular scheme in tough times.[22] While this did correspond with a period of Labour control, support extended beyond party lines. The Liberal local newspaper, the *Barnsley Chronicle*, for example, ran an editorial in 1926 which simply stated that:

21 See (all from the *Barnsley Chronicle*) 'Barnsley County Borough Council', 18 June 1921; 'Protest against Ministry's Act', 15 October 1921; 'Items from the Minutes', 17 December 1921. The Ministry had proposed restricting the grant for the provision of free milk to 5 per cent of costs, but Barnsley was successful in campaigning for the original 50 per cent contribution.

22 'Milk for Infants', *Barnsley Chronicle*, 24 July 1926.

> [i]t is a widely know axiom that healthy infancy presupposes an abundance of wholesome milk ... The quibble by the Ministry of Health [over the supplementary grant] was very properly brushed aside by the Council, who approved of the Medical Officer's action in continuing the supply of milk. The health and robustness of the rising generation in Barnsley are manifestly of far more vital importance to the community than the 'anise and cumin' of Whitehall's bureaucratic regulation.[23]

From 1926 until the end of the interwar period milk provision continued to increase dramatically; with the exception of the period of Independent control of the council in 1931. Not only did spending reduce then, but the council appears to have tightened up their policing of the scheme as part of a more general economy drive.[24] From the time that the Labour Party regained full control of the council in 1933, until 1939, free milk provision rocketed, indicating the level of political commitment to what was effectively a stigma-free benefit subsidy.[25]

Outside this scheme, Labour's influence on MCW services was diluted by wider questions of finance and the integration of healthcare provision in the borough. A plan for a new maternity home, for example, was held up while the future of the transferred institution was debated (as is discussed in greater detail below), and it was not built until 1937–8.[26] The greatest expansion both in expenditure and services did take place during the period of Labour control in the 1930s, however, for example the opening of a long-planned new infant welfare centre (in 1935), the reorganisation of the health visitor scheme, and the appointment of a new Assistant MOH and nurse to serve the new clinic.[27] The council also reduced fees for necessitous cases,

23 'Barnsley Municipal Topics', *Barnsley Chronicle*, 31 July 1926.

24 See for example BALS Minutes of Barnsley County Borough Council, Public Health Services Committee Minutes, 1 May 1931 for instances of the committee prosecuting individuals for falsely claiming that they had an entitlement to free milk.

25 This subsidy was particularly necessary given the low levels of female participation in the workforce, and the large average family size.

26 'Barnsley's New Civic Head Elected', *Barnsley Chronicle*, 13 November 1937. This was despite the hospital being appropriated in 1936, and improvements being made to the maternity wards.

27 The new centre was first discussed in 1924, when the existing facilities were criticised by the Ministry of Health. See BALS: Minutes of Barnsley County Borough Council,

and extended the maternity services available in the borough.[28] This was part of a Labour campaign to reduce the high maternal mortality, which by the early 1930s was double the national average.[29] The Independents had made only limited responses to a 1931 Ministry memo on the subject, but the Labour Party stated unequivocally that 'health ought to come first and expense afterwards', and moved rapidly on the Ministry's recommendations once they were back in power in 1933.[30] The maternal mortality rate subsequently fell dramatically, and by mid-decade was well under the national level; a reversal of trend which was taken by the Labour controlled council as an endorsement of their efforts.[31] Barnsley also formed a domiciliary midwife service in accordance with the 1936 Midwives Act which was part of the (by then) integrated maternity services of the town.[32]

Maternity and Child Welfare Committee Minutes, 3 March and 1 December 1924; 'Barnsley inspects new clinic', *Barnsley Chronicle*, 25 January 1936; TNA MH66/1066, Survey Report, Barnsley, 86–7.

28 See BALS: Minutes of Barnsley County Borough Council, Public Health Services Committee Minutes, 30 December 1932, 28 July 1933, 4 January 1935, 28 June 1935.

29 Annual Returns on Maternal Mortality, Annual Report of the Chief Medical Officer (London, 1930–8), Appendix C.

30 'High Infant Mortality', *Barnsley Chronicle*, 12 September 1931. The measures which were passed by the Independent-controlled council in 1931 included setting aside £50 to pay consultants to advise and treat abnormal cases; the borough engineer and the MOH were to report on proposals to enlarge the maternity home; and an amount not exceeding £10 was allotted for buying sterilised maternity outfits for selected cases ('Maternal Mortality', *Barnsley Chronicle*, 17 October 1931).

31 In 1935 Councillor Jones argued in his budget speech that the sharp reduction in the maternal mortality rate justified the increase in the rates. See 'My Budget', *Barnsley Chronicle*, 16 March 1935. According to the Annual Returns of the Registrar General, the mortality per thousand 'in the puerperal state' (sepsis and other) fell from 9.7 in 1931 to 3 in 1935 in Barnsley, although it had been significantly lower in 1930 (3.4). The national rates in the same years were both 4.4. Barnsley fell below the national rate for the first time since 1930 in 1933 (Reports of the Registrar General, 1931–5). In 1933 Sheerien had also stated in council that the Public Health Committee 'were not looking at the matter [of funding midwives] from a financial point of view, but from the point of view of maternal mortality and with a view to decreasing it in Barnsley.' 'Barnsley Borough Council', *Barnsley Chronicle*, 14 January 1933.

32 The nine municipal midwives were to deal with 640 of the 1890 births in the town annually. The remainder were managed at the expanded maternity home at the

The MCW services clearly illustrate the impact of Labour's prioritising of ameliorative health schemes, although it is also apparent that some of their improvements were built on earlier policies. In the 1920s the schemes under this head in Barnsley were limited and underfunded, with political support only strongly and consistently behind the provision of free milk to necessitous women. This initiative accounted almost entirely for the high levels of expenditure per head on MCW services. Greater Labour representation, together with a strong push from the Ministry survey and the maternal mortality studies (and also a more sympathetic MOH, Dr Scott, in the key years 1932–5) all then prompted a marked change in the level and quality of the town's provision for mothers and children. By the late 1930s Barnsley's health department had developed and was trying to implement a comprehensive and long term approach to maternity care, which contained scope for future.[33] The first period of Labour control also saw the council making full declarations under the 1929 Local Government Act, and the second, the appropriation of the transferred institution, both of which also affected the delivery of the MCW schemes. It is to this attempt to coordinate the entire health services of the borough which we now turn.

The Labour Party and Appropriation

Barnsley was the only one of our case study boroughs to appropriate its transferred institution, Gawber Road Infirmary (renamed St Helen's Hospital after appropriation in April 1936). In the early 1930s the Infirmary

appropriated PAI, the private nursing home, and by private midwives. This allowed for better co-ordination and higher standards, supported by more up-to-date equipment. See MOH, Annual Report, Barnsley, 1936, p. 105.

33 In 1937 the MOH gave an outline of recommendations to further reduce the maternal mortality rate, which had risen again in that year. This included a range of self-help measures to improve diet and general health, and council support in the form of an enlarged maternity hospital and Emergency Maternity Service. MOH, Annual Report, Barnsley, 1937, p. 17.

and PAI together had a total of 490 beds, of which 236 were on the House (Public Assistance) side. This included a limited amount of specialised accommodation: a four-bed maternity ward, with attached labour ward; ten beds in the male TB ward; two two-bedded open air shelters, and twenty beds (ten each male and female) in three wards for VD, scabies and 'other unpleasant cases.' These, however, might also be used for overflow from the mental wards.[34] The West Riding County Council retained user-ship rights to the accommodation, although two thirds of the beds were reserved for Barnsley patients.

The Labour council was prompt to make extensive declarations about its plan to run the hospital under Public Health rather than Public Assistance schemes, although the actual improvements took longer to put in place.[35] As early as April 1930, the Chair of the new PAC, the Labour councillor Joseph Jones, stated that they had the intention of turning the infirmary into a 'a public hospital in the greater sense', and to better co-ordinate the hospital facilities in the borough. The intention towards social levelling and widening citizenship in these sentiments was clear – better co-ordination of maternity services with the voluntary Beckett Hospital was desired, for example: 'so that it could not be said of any citizen in the future that he or she had been born in the workhouse ... A very grave responsibility had been placed upon the [the council], and in the future it would be their duty to compensate for the inequalities of nature's endowments, and handicaps of adversity'.[36]

The first step on this road was taken when the Labour-dominated council cut the ties between the Poor Law and the new Public Assistance Committee, by refusing to allow any of the ex-Guardians positions on the

34 TNA MH66/1066, Survey Report, Barnsley, 152–4.

35 The original declarations were withdrawn while the ownership of the institution was disputed between the County Borough and the County Council. Barnsley subsequently submitted reworked declarations which stated their intention 'as soon as circumstances permit' to provide all possible services under acts other than Poor Law. TNA MH66/1066, Survey Report, Barnsley, 148–50.

36 'Poor Law Relief – The New PAC Meets', *Barnsley Chronicle*, 12 April 1930.

Committee.[37] A similarly symbolic break with the past was made with the renaming of the hospital on its eventual appropriation.[38]

The plans for appropriation and improvement stalled somewhat during the early 1930s, and patients were not all redirected to treatment under the public health schemes.[39] The delay was partly the result of wrangling with the County Council, plus the change in control of the council in November 1931 to the more economically minded Independents, and then to a hung council between 1932 and 1933. This was the situation at the time of the Ministry survey of the state of the health services since the Local Government Act. The plans were also held up because of tensions between the several medical officers and committees involved, which will be detailed further below and which were also a central feature of West Hartlepool's debates regarding appropriation. By the time that Labour regained control in November 1933 all that had been done officially by the council was the formation of a Joint Advisory Committee to consider the whole question of the PAI's future.[40] Despite this, the Town Clerk had informed the Ministry inspector in 1932 that: 'he could take it that it is the Council's desire to carry out, so far as possible, the principles of the Local Government Act, 1929, with regard to the transfer of services from Poor Law administration'.[41]

The case for appropriation was lent weight by the support of the Ministry of Health. Its survey report in 1932 did not give a very promising picture of the accommodation in the ex-workhouse part of the institution, but it recommended the appropriation of the medical parts and the development of a number of different services to be based there. This would also

37 In contrast, in West Hartlepool the continued dominance of the old Poor Law Guardians on the PAC was one of the key factors in ensuring the non-appropriation of Howbeck PAI.

38 See A. Levene, 'Between Less Eligibility and the NHS: The Changing Place of Poor Law Hospitals in England and Wales, 1929–39', *Twentieth Century British History*, 20:3 (2009).

39 TNA MH66/420, Survey Report Appendices, Barnsley, Appendix O, 150–1.

40 Ibid.

41 TNA MH66/1066, Survey Report, Barnsley, 150–1.

ease demand at the voluntary Beckett Hospital, where there were waiting lists for admission, thus making 'the two hospitals mutually auxiliary and not competitive'.[42] In order to bring Gawber Road up to the standard of a general hospital the inspector recommended extending the staff accommodation, and building some new infrastructure, including patient lifts, an operating theatre, an X-ray department and a small laboratory.[43]

When in 1934 the Labour Party again dominated the council (with a majority of eight) they quickly demonstrated that they were keen to move forward on the issue of appropriation. They published a plan of action for the town which prioritised '[i]mproved social services as a whole, but with a stabilised rate in the £'. A key part of this programme was the 'coordination of the whole town's hospital services', which included appropriating the Infirmary part of the PAI and improving cooperation between it and the voluntary Beckett Hospital.[44] The Labour Mayor, Councillor Jones, again made the intentions of his Party and of the council very clear, stating that: 'it is hoped that [the new municipal hospital] will be utilised to the full and be a boon to the citizens of the town. The whole project to appropriation

42 These included maternity services, adenoidal and tonsil operations for children, inpatient treatment for orthopaedic patients, and for VD. The part of the Ministry's report dealing with the voluntary Beckett Hospital noted that almost all tonsil and adenoid cases had to be treated as outpatients because of lack of space on the wards. The X-ray department was also insufficient at the voluntary hospital. The Ministry inspector envisaged that the major surgical cases would be treated at the Beckett, and that the municipal hospital be recognised as a training centre for nurses. TNA MH66/1066, Survey Report, Barnsley, 157–60 and 166–7, and TNA MH66/420, Survey Report Appendices, Barnsley, Appendix O.10, Local Government Act, 1929, Some points for consideration in Barnsley.

43 TNA MH66/1066, Survey Report, Barnsley, 157–9.

44 'Labour Plans', *Barnsley Chronicle*, 24 November 1934. The judgement of the wards at the Beckett Hospital was mixed, and varied according to their age: '[t]he medical wards struck me as somewhat overcrowded, but the newer wards have ample space, light and ventilation, and are very satisfactory.' Ministry of Health Survey Report, Barnsley, p. 165. The 149 beds were made up of 16 medical, 60 surgical, 16 orthopaedic, 15 eye, 12 gynaecological, 2 maternity, 1 for sick staff, and 27 children.

is to provide for the more efficient hospital treatment of the sick, and to divorce, as far as possible, this treatment from the Poor Law.'[45]

Similarly, the Chair of the PAC said that he was 'interested in the appropriation because he saw it as a step towards the provision of a higher and more efficient standard of service.'[46] It is perhaps worth noting here that while the Labour Party self-consciously styled their plans in terms of socialist priorities, appropriation of itself was not necessarily a political issue. The 1929 Act had, after all, been promoted by the Conservative Neville Chamberlain and in London the Municipal Reform Party – effectively the Conservatives – took a positive stance towards appropriation.[47] This is in marked contrast with Eastbourne where there did not seem to be such a clear rationale behind the pro-appropriation sentiment.

Gawber Road Infirmary officially became St Helen's appropriated general hospital in 1936, and plans continued to raise medical and staffing standards, and improve the general atmosphere of the institution.[48] A Resident Medical Officer was also appointed for the first time in the hospital's history, and he (and his successor) was a further force for improvement.[49] Progress towards better co-ordination of hospital services in the borough was slower than first anticipated, but by March 1937 the Public Health Committee (PHC) had drawn up a plan of management. This included the sharing of new services and consultant staff, a division of the case load between the municipal and voluntary hospitals (chronic, many of the

45 'Antidote to Last Year's Budget Shock', *Barnsley Chronicle*, 14 March 1936.

46 'Appropriation of Institution Hospital', *Barnsley Chronicle*, 14 March 1936.

47 See Stewart, '"The Finest Municipal Hospital Service in the World'.

48 This included, for example, making a largely symbolic fence divide between the new hospital and the PAI, and giving the hospital nurses new uniforms. Larger improvements consisted of a new nurses' home, modernisation of some of the wards and infrastructure, and the building of a new maternity block with twenty beds.

49 The first Medical Officer was Dr William Simpson, formerly the Senior Assistant Medical Officer at St Alfege's Hospital in London, one of the largest PAIs appropriated by the London County Council (MOH Annual Report, Barnsley, 1936, p. 30). He was succeeded in the following year by Dr Isaac Rose, who had previously worked as Resident Surgical Officer at Barnsley's Beckett Hospital, and briefly as Assistant Surgeon to the LCC ('St Helen Hospital', *Barnsley Chronicle*, 12 June 1937).

acute medical, a small number of acute surgical cases at St Helen's); and joint meetings to co-ordinate work.[50] Attempts to integrate the municipal maternity services between St Helen's and the new maternity home were a long time coming, as we have already noted, but had largely been achieved by the end of our period.[51]

We do not have any records which reveal how straightforward it was to come to these arrangements between the municipal and voluntary sectors, but it is reasonable to suggest that the process was eased by the fact that many Labour men sat as miners' representatives on the Beckett Hospital Committee. The popular Beckett Hospital received most of its funding for annual expenditure from contributory and work schemes, so it was also closely associated with the interests of the largest socio-economic and occupational groups in the town.[52] Indeed, it was the only voluntary organisation in Barnsley to be well supported, in contrast with the situation in Newport, our other Labour-influenced case study. This popular support from the working classes (who were the principal users of the hospital)

50 'Hospital Services Coordination', *Barnsley Chronicle*, 13 March 1937. St Helen's was also to deal with some fracture cases, obstetrical cases, with a certain amount of gynaecological work, in-patient treatment of ophthalmia neonatorum, X-ray work, and routine dental work for their own inpatients. The shared services included a new pathological service based at St Helen's.

51 For example, the popular Medical Officer there, Dr Rose, encouraged mothers to immunise their babies, and an emergency maternity service and facilities to treat opthalmia neonatorum were provided. MOH Annual Report, Barnsley, 1936, Report of St Helen Hospital by Dr Simpson, 123–4. By 1938 there were four times as many maternity cases at the appropriated hospital as in 1936, and there was much better communication between services. There were no deaths under the new system in 1938 (MOH Annual Report, Barnsley, 1938, pp. 1 & 3).

52 The hospital was able to pay off its £20,000 post-war debt within six months, for example, thanks to an appeal from the Miners' Public Hall. It was also supported by the Saturday and Sunday Fund Committee, the Barnsley British Co-operative Society and a few local gentry ('Out for £20,000', *Barnsley Chronicle*, 21 February 1920 and 'Lady Sutherland and the Beckett Hospital', *Barnsley Chronicle*, 29 October 1921). The Miners' Welfare Fund also paid for a new outpatient department in 1929, with a large waiting area, consulting and dressing rooms, X-ray and massage departments. 'Hospital Conference', *Barnsley Chronicle*, 30 March 1929.

demonstrates a real cultural difference from some other boroughs where voluntary institutions received most of their support from 'the great and the good'. The Beckett Hospital was thus tied directly to popular interests to a much greater extent than its equivalent in Newport, for example. Given that, in Barnsley, the popular interest which sat on the board of the Beckett Hospital was also that which influenced the leaders of the council, links with the municipal service were much more likely, and likely to succeed than elsewhere.

There were still tensions in later years – for example, in 1938 a non-Labour councillor demanded that the long-standing annual grant of £500 from the council to the Beckett be stopped – but on the whole, the Labour council felt that its efforts to improve co-ordination of hospital-based services in the borough had been a success. In 1937 the new Labour Mayor, Alderman Wright, was reported in the *Barnsley Chronicle* as saying that '[a]t the St Helen Hospital the transformation is quietly taking place from a grim Poor Law Hospital to that of a modern hospital supplying the medical needs of the inhabitants.'[53] Admissions figures bear out the Mayor's words: in the first full year following appropriation, there was a 42 per cent increase in admissions (from 741 in 1936 to 1052 in 1937). This was accompanied by a 'welcome change' in the type of patient, with fewer senile and chronic cases and increase in acute medical cases.[54] Despite this, further plans were held back by the need for economy (for example, the shortage of beds for mental health patients could not be addressed), and by the outbreak of the war the hospital was still in part being held back by its poor law roots. The MOH recognised this in 1938, but also the strong commitment to improvement from the council:

> It is sometimes stated that the 'stigma' which attached the hospital in the past when it belonged to the sphere of [the] Poor Law might remain, but I am sure that the new better services which the Hospital sub-Committee are determined to provide will move such a feeling. There are limitations of course in the type and design of the building, its external appearance, and many failings in the interior construction

53 'Barnsley's New Civic Head Elected', *Barnsley Chronicle*, 13 November 1937.

54 See Levene, 'Between less eligibility'.

> of the building, but no effort will be spared by the whole staff of the Public Health Department which serves the St Helen Hospital to bring this hospital up to first class standard, which will compare with any of the splendid hospitals of whatever type throughout the country. Such is our determination, and I am proud of the consideration which the Committee gives to the improvement of the hospital.[55]

The concerted effort to improve and expand hospital services demonstrates again Labour's commitment to improving municipal services, and the articulate way that they expressed their aims links this overtly to their social vision for the borough.[56] While there were other significant factors shaping health services in Barnsley, some of which we expand on in the subsequent section, the underlying rationale for improved municipal provision while Labour was in control is plain. As the MCW schemes also showed, the pace of investment and reform dwindled under the economy-minded Independents, and while Labour's voice was restrained on the hung councils of the early 1930s, their efforts were visible again almost immediately after they retook control in 1933. The support of the Ministry of Health undoubtedly also lent weight to their campaign, but perhaps the strongest evidence of the link between the shape of the health services and the Labour Party in this borough is offered in a speech by the Labour mayor in 1938: 'Our health services today are, indeed, a triumph of municipal progress, and every year one is impressed by their constant expansion; through the medium of local government, expert attention is no longer the especial privilege of any particular class'.[57]

55 MOH Annual Report, Barnsley, 1938, pp. 31–2.

56 It was also party policy by this stage. See Stewart, *The Battle for Health*.

57 'Cllr Cassells Eighth Labour Mayor of Barnsley', *Barnsley Chronicle*, 12 November 1938.

Non-Labour Influences on Health

The Labour Party in Barnsley had an unarguably large role in shaping the form and pace of investment in the health services in the latter part of the interwar period. We have already noted, however, that many of their plans had roots in the 1920s or earlier, or were priorities that crossed party lines. This warns against placing too much weight on party as an explanatory factor, although it should be remembered that Barnsley had a significantly higher proportion of Labour councillors even in the 1920s than most other boroughs. This, and the strong influence of trade unions and the co-operative movement probably influenced spending decisions before Labour controlled the council. The free milk scheme is one example, and the generous allowance for extra nourishment for tuberculous patients in the 1920s is another.[58] In other cases, however, Labour was unable to make further headway because of other influences in the borough: the financial caution of the Independents, for example; the attitude of the MOH or other medical officers; the nature of relationships between other parties; or the position taken by the Ministry of Health (whose sanction was necessary for loans).

The borough's poor financial position was one of the biggest constraints on the development of the municipal services, and one which affected the attitude of the Ministry of Health to expansion as well. It affected the length of time it took for the medical services clinic to be built, for example; it limited the extensions and improvements at the hospitals and TB sanatorium, including the opening of new maternity facilities; and it had an impact also on the fund-raising efforts of the voluntary Beckett Hospital. In addition, it resulted in the Ministry of Health being unwilling

58 BALS: Minutes of Barnsley County Borough Council, Barnsley Treatment of Tuberculosis Committee minutes, 8 June 1921.The council chose to allow the maximum amount possible. Other significant expansions were made to the TB services in the 1920s, including the expansion of the sanatorium and the provision of new clinics and treatments (BALS: Minutes of Barnsley County Borough Council, Medical Services Committee minutes, 6 December 1926, 31 January 1927, 2 May 1927 and 30 May 1927).

to sanction expenditure, even when it admitted that it was necessary. However, the impact of the economic situation was probably exaggerated by the change in control of the council towards the Independents from November 1930 to 1932, and the fact that Labour did not fully regain control until November 1933. The dip in spending in these years is probably the result of the combination of the two factors, rather than the impact of economic problems alone.

Finance was also a big issue in the relationship between the Ministry of Health and Barnsley council, particularly during the years of Labour control. As one Ministry of Health official put it '[t]his is a somewhat difficult authority with which to deal. They have a fair standard of progress in health work, but their financial position is serious and they are rather given to making expensive proposals for capital expenditure without full consideration of the need ...'[59]

The Ministry recognised that the borough had a desperate need for better health services, but as one official noted in an internal minute of 1935, 'I feel some doubt whether, in view of the parlous state of Barnsley's finances, it will be possible to permit of this expenditure [on capital projects], *although it cannot be said that any of it is unnecessary*' [emphasis added].[60] This tendency to rein in the borough's more expansive plans dates back into the 1920s as well, when the Ministry limited the grant to underwrite the provision of free milk, and refused to subsidise buying the land for the MCW clinic. While sympathetic to the tension between medical need and poor finances, Whitehall felt the need to offer a restraining hand to what they saw as excessiveness: 'They have quite run riot in proposals for nurses' accommodation ... The council seem to want to blame the Ministry for holding up proposals for development, but we must see the necessity for such heavy expenditure is justified.'[61]

59 TNA MH66/421, Survey Correspondence, Barnsley, Minute by Ministry of Health Official Ward, 8 November 1934. The financial returns used in this study exclude capital expenditure, although the figures are available.

60 Ibid. Minute by Farrow, 16 July 1935.The plan involved capital expenditure of £46,000. It included a new nurses' home (£22,000), a medical superintendent's house, a children's home, a mortuary, boiler, fence, and building for mental defectives (£10,000).

61 Ibid. Minute by Ministry of Health official Ward, 8 November 1934.

This attitude was tempered when it came to the improvements required at St Helen's Hospital following appropriation, where the Ministry recognised that certain costs would be 'very considerable' but necessary. Nonetheless, officials wondered 'whether the Council can be allowed to go on with these proposals.'[62] Although the Minister did give his consent to appropriation, and agreed the building of a maternity unit was 'a matter of urgent necessity,' he urged that 'in view of the financial circumstances of the borough' other improvements must be considered in relation to the 'urgency of need and the estimated cost.'[63] All the suggested improvements were ones recommended by the Ministry's own inspector, but this did not override the eye to the financial balance sheet when the prospect of paying for them arose. This delayed the expansion and co-ordination of the institutional maternity services for a number of years.

The financial situation of the town took a turn for the worse in 1935 when the District Auditor reported a number of financial irregularities. Not only had a revenue deficiency built up, but Sinking Fund money had also been kept in hand rather than being invested or used to pay debts. There was also 'persistent overspending,' and Reserve Funds and balances were 'raided to relieve the rates.' This further inclined the Ministry to refuse to sanction additional loans, and this was reinforced when the costs of raising nurses' salaries was revealed in 1935.[64] The council was forced to review their finances, which they did in a marathon session in 1937. One of the results was the suspension of the much vaunted forty-hour week, which as well as being a job creation scheme, had significantly reduced the working hours of the nursing staff. A supplementary rate of 4/3d in the pound also had to be levied, bringing the total rates to 22/5d, although the motion to permanently abandon the forty-hour week was ultimately defeated.[65]

The Labour Mayor, however, argued that the present crisis was the result of the financial culture before his party took control in 1928:

62 Ibid. Letter from Farrow to Neville, 15 December 1934. These included building a new porter's lodge and fence to divide the hospital from the House; patient lifts and an operating theatre, staff accommodation and a maternity block.

63 Ibid. Letter from Ministry of Health to Barnsley, 25 June 1935.

64 Ibid. Letter from Ministry of Health to Barnsley, 13 August 1935.

65 'A 40-Hour Week Experiment,' *Northern Daily Mail*, 2 April 1937.

'a legacy of administrative confusion and financial embarrassment, inevitably calculated in due time to create a condition of quasi-insolvency'.[66] Furthermore, he declared that the Independent administration had operated with a 'cowardly disregard for the future' passing on debts of nearly £3.5million and annual loan charges of £239,834. Speaking against him in the council debate, Councillor Soper described the forty-hour week policy as an 'orgy of recklessness'.[67] Nonetheless, there was a strong tendency from the Council to see the Ministry of Health as unnecessarily obstructive to what they saw as vital improvements.

This inability to balance the vision for a comprehensive, good quality health service with the realities of the financial situation really characterises the wider context in Barnsley. Their financial irregularities indicate that the council was not administering their finances correctly, but there was no suggestion of wrongdoing. Rather, they were using funds in order to try and develop their services. This suggests that the block grant was failing in its purpose of redistributing wealth to the neediest areas, and that necessary reform was stymied to a certain extent by financial resources. The financial situation also made the Ministry of Health chary of allowing even necessary investment, which was a further brake on the coherent development of good services, and one which the council resented. Like Barnsley itself, Whitehall lacked the funds to permit large-scale expenditure, which is what the Labour council was inclined to promote.

Amidst all these discussions and tensions, the Medical Officers of Health played a relatively small role. This contrasts particularly with the influence of the strong-minded and well connected MOH in Eastbourne, Dr William Willoughby. In Barnsley the role of the MOHs was downplayed, partly because there was quite a high turnover of officers (six during the interwar period), but also perhaps because the need to push an expan-

66 'Barnsley New Rate of 18/9 Levied at Marathon Council sitting,' *Barnsley Chronicle*, 17 April 1937. The council sat for seven hours, with one twenty minute break, to listen to and debate this budget speech.

67 'Barnsley New Rate of 18/9 Levied at Marathon Council sitting,' *Barnsley Chronicle*, 17 April 1937.

sionist agenda was removed by the coterminous attitude of the council.[68] The various Medical Officers of Health were generally in favour of progressive schemes like the appropriation of Gawber Road PAI, and the expansion of the MCW services, but they offered little in the way of significant leadership. Indeed, the MOH at the time of the Local Government Act managed to offend the PAC to the extent that they would only allow him to come to their meetings when specifically invited.[69] The standing and dynamism of the council's chief medical representatives may also have been affected by the low salary compared with other County Boroughs; a situation which Labour was averse to changing despite their support of salary raises for nurses and health visitors.[70] In a borough less motivated to expand services some of the Medical Officers of Health might have

68 None of the Medical Officers of Health seem to have been overtly Labour men, although Lindley notes that nationally some Party members advocated that sympathetic officers be appointed to local councils (Lindley, 'The Party Machine', 45). He also suggests that this happened in Barnsley 'to a small degree', but it must have been through more distant connections, since all of the medical officers were out-of-town appointments.

69 The situation arose because the then MOH, Dr MacDonald, had asked for an increase in salary on becoming the Medical Officer to the PAC. The Medical Officer at Gawber Road was affronted and became sensitive to any suggestion that MacDonald was 'meddling' at the institution. As a result, neither he nor his successor had free access to patients there. See TNA MH66/1066, Survey Report, Barnsley, 147–8.

70 Labour's reasons for opposing raising the MOH's salary were the need for economy ('Medical Officer's Salary Increase Opposed,' *Barnsley Chronicle*, 17 January 1925). The MOH's salary was not increased until 1936 (to £1000 per annum), when he also became Medical Superintendant of St Helen's Hospital. Even then, the final level was still only the minimum *starting* salary recommended by the BMA for Medical Officers of Health in towns the size of Barnsley since the early 1920s. Both West Hartlepool and Newport paid their MOHs at a higher level than Barnsley (Teesside Archives CB/WH/C2/179, West Hartlepool Health Committee Minutes, 1919 to 1937, 25 November 1929, extract from the Minutes of the Council of the Association of Municipal Corporations, 17 October 1929). The Town Clerk had also resigned in 1920 because of his low salary compared with other boroughs. See 'Town Clerk of Barnsley,' *Barnsley Chronicle*, 22 May 1920 and 'Town Clerk to Resign,' *Barnsley Chronicle*, 12 June 1920.

played a bigger part in shaping policies, but in Barnsley the problem seems to have been restraining plans for expansion rather than instigating them, and the Medical Officers of Health generally took a supporting rather than a leading role.

Other plans for reform were affected by tensions between different committees and personnel. Altercations between the PHC and the Education Committee held up plans for a new joint infant welfare clinic which had been first proposed in 1924, for example, and which was approved by the Ministry of Health in 1932.[71] It was not until the summer of 1933 that both the Board of Education and the Ministry of Health fully approved the clinic because of lack of agreement over funding and services, and it opened in November of 1935.[72] Plans to expand the Kendray infectious disease hospital proposed in 1924 became mired in disputes between Barnsley and the surrounding Urban and Rural District Councils who used it. Five years of disputes ensued, during which time several of the out-districts broke off and attempted to form their own isolation hospital in order to escape what they saw as the dominating attitudes of Barnsley County Borough. A full agreement was not reached with the out-districts until 1935, when permanent extensions could finally be built.[73] Disputes like this between bodies with different priorities and demands were typical of municipal politics in all four of our case studies.

71 'Over £10,000 for a New Clinic', *Barnsley Chronicle*, 14 May 1932. The Ministry's Survey Report noted that the plans were still being held up by the Education Committee (TNA MH66/1066, Survey Report, Barnsley, 82–3).

72 BALS Minutes of Barnsley County Borough Council, Public Health Services Committee minutes, 26 May 1933. The general strike and the depression had also played a part in the delays.

73 A temporary block had been built in 1929, but accommodation for diphtheria and scarlet fever epidemics in 1928 and 1929 had been problematic.

Conclusions

The discussion of Barnsley County Borough has demonstrated that it fulfils its characterisation as a poor, high spending, and Labour-dominated town. It has illustrated the positive impact that the Labour Party could have on investment in health, and in this borough this is very clearly linked with party sentiment. Our second Labour case study, Newport, will indicate that this was not always so forcefully the case. However, there was more to spending levels than simply party colour: the Labour Party in Barnsley was strongly influenced by trade unions and the co-operative movement, and this shaped the attitude to services generally and the strength the Party had behind it. These bodies were also well represented at the voluntary Beckett Hospital, so that while the voluntary sector generally was less well developed than in other towns, this institution had much support from people also involved in council business. This eased good relations between the institutions after 1929. The Labour inclination to spend was not universal either; witness the reluctance to raise the salary of the MOH, although this can be linked to class-based ideals (and prejudices). Certainly the Labour Party was forceful in raising the salaries and benefits of nurses and health visitors, and instituting the forty-hour week for council staff. There is also evidence to suggest that the council sometimes came up with schemes which the Ministry of Health saw as profligate and unnecessary, however: an inclination to spend did not necessarily correlate with well judged services.

These inclinations were also significantly reined in in Barnsley because of its poor financial situation. This was inherent to the poor rateable value of the borough, high rates notwithstanding, although it is significant that the problem was not particularly eased by the introduction of the block grant in 1929. The town had considerable need of good health services: its housing was poor and overcrowded, it had high maternal mortality for part of the period, and its environment was polluted. Its chief employment sector was also impoverished and unstable by this period. Yet it was unable to meet all these demands because of its straitened finances; a situation which was exacerbated by unwise manipulation of its finances. This resulted in the Ministry of Health's refusal to sanction several loans; setbacks which the council felt were unmerited.

Infighting on the council, and troubled relations with other authorities and sectors did play a part in Barnsley, but not to the extent seen in some of our other case studies. Nor were individuals on the council committees (outside the Labour leadership) as influential as they were, for example, in Eastbourne. Overall, we may characterise Barnsley as a town with a genuine commitment to developing high quality health services, with an inclination to spend beyond its means, and very limited funds with which to work. This situation characterises most of the interwar period, but there is no doubt that it was magnified in the years of Labour control. This was made overtly clear in their own statements. In 1938 the *Barnsley Chronicle* reported the view of Labour councillors that money spent on the health services was

> the best investment the Council could make, and figures which could be produced to show an improvement in the health of the people, clearly proved that what had been spent on medical services had been the very best investment the council had ever made. With reference to other towns ... [it was] a mistake to base their policy on other places. There might be some, but [they] did not know of any that could show a better record than Barnsley with regard to medical services.[74]

74 'Medical Appointment Protest,' *Barnsley Chronicle*, 16 July 1938.

CHAPTER FIVE

Eastbourne

Eastbourne, our second case study, stands in marked contrast with Barnsley in almost every respect: wealthy, southern, healthy, with the distinctive social and employment profile of a resort town, and very low levels of Labour involvement on the council. Eastbourne has long been known as a well-off resort on the south coast, with a high proportion of retired residents, and a distinctly middle-class profile. In the interwar period this was reflected in the high proportion of domestic servants in its population, low levels of crowding, a high average age and a low birth rate. Ministry of Health inspectors visiting the borough in 1933 noted the affluent nature of the town, and its good climate. They described the housing as 'reasonably good,' with a below average percentage of families living more than two persons to a room, and few unfit houses. The main industry of the town was tourism and its attractions as a 'health resort' meant that it had a significant, and affluent, visitor population. It also had a reputation for its schooling, with one public school, twenty-one boys' preparatory schools, and eighteen schools for girls, all housing a total of three thousand boarders, as well as numerous day schools.[1]

Financially, the borough was relatively well off. Unemployment was low; by some way the lowest of any of the four case studies. Even in the 1930s, when rising levels of joblessness made themselves felt even in this well-off borough, rates were still only just over half the County Borough average – 7 per cent of the adult male population in 1931 compared to 16

1 TNA MH66/1071, Survey Report, Eastbourne, 1–2; Census of England and Wales, 1921 and 1931.

per cent across the dataset nationally.[2] This relatively protected position meant that even during the straitened early thirties the council was able to keep the rates low compared with other boroughs and the national average, and they remained low even when rates had a hike nationally after the 1929 Local Government Act. This in turn was eased by the high rateable value of the property base, on which taxation revenue was based: this was double the national average from 1929, and still substantially above the average before that as well (see Figures 3.7b and e in Chapter Three).

The borough was thus able to support spending on its municipal services without putting an undue burden on its ratepayers, and the council took it as a point of pride to make good provision for healthcare. This was partly in response to the needs of its high-profile elderly population, but it was also designed to project a good outward image to visitors.[3] The town supported a large and active medical profession, and an abnormally large number of hospitals. In fact, this commitment to hospitals and other institutions is one of the most distinctive characteristics of Eastbourne's health provision across both municipal and voluntary sectors. Where most towns might support one voluntary hospital, Eastbourne sustained six, the largest being the Princess Alice Memorial Hospital, with 110 beds.[4] It also had numerous nursing homes, a TB hospital (Gildredge), an infectious diseases hospital, a smallpox hospital, a maternity home and from 1930 St Mary's, the ex-Poor Law institution, all under municipal control. This

2 Census, 1931. This figure does not include retired males. The Ministry of Health surveyor quoted a rate of 12.7 per cent in Eastbourne compared with 24.4 per cent nationally (TNA MH66/1071, Survey Report, Eastbourne, 3).

3 In 1932 the MOH attributed the lack of reduction in death rates locally to the aging population of the town (MOH Annual Report, Eastbourne, 1932, vii). He also attributed a rise in TB rates in the early 1920s to a large number of visitors coming to the town for the sake of their health (MOH Annual Report, Eastbourne, 1921, pp. 43 & 48). Cancer rates were also high.

4 The others were The Royal Eye Hospital, The Ear Nose and Throat Hospital, All Saints Hospital (for women and children), the Leaf Homeopathic Cottage Hospital and The London Homeopathic Hospital Convalescent Unit. Taken from J. Clarke, *History of the Eastbourne Medical Society, 1883–1983* (Eastbourne, 1983), Appendix 4. See below for more details on the voluntary hospitals.

was for a town with a population which scarcely exceeded 60,000 in 1921, and contracted somewhat thereafter.[5] As in Newport, the voluntary sector had a prominent profile, but in Eastbourne, the particular preference for institutions was continued into the municipal arena as well.

This brief picture thus confirms that Eastbourne was a wealthy borough, and also one with quite distinctive social and economic characteristics. Figure 5.1 illustrates that it also conforms to its typology as a high spender on health services compared with the national picture, at least until 1935.[6] In contrast to most other boroughs, there was no strong upward trend in spending over the interwar period, but this can largely be accounted for by its early generosity. This meant that its advantage over other boroughs was gradually eroded, however, as they stepped up their investment in health services and it did not. In 1922 Eastbourne spent almost double the County Borough average of £334 per thousand on health, but by 1935 the gap between its expenditure of £661 per thousand and the much raised national figure of £513 was significantly reduced. In fact in the following year expenditure in Eastbourne dropped sharply for the first time in the interwar period, and fell below the average expenditure per thousand. The reasons behind this abrupt change of trend will be explored in greater detail below. Unfortunately we lack figures on spending after 1936, but other evidence on council debates suggest that 1935 marked the beginning of an unwillingness to spend and invest in health services in the town.

5 The population of Eastbourne was recorded at 62,028 in the 1921 census, and 57.435 in 1931. See also Chapter 3, Figure 3.7a.

6 See Chapter 3, Figure 3.7d for a comparison with the other case studies.

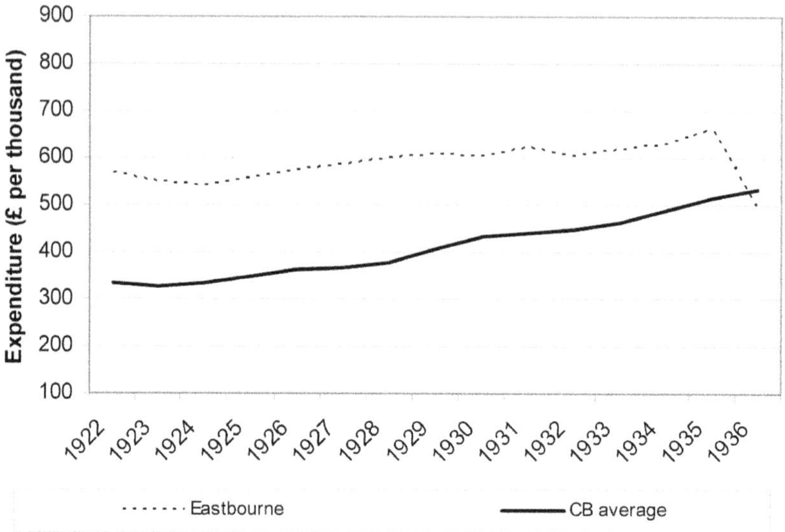

Figure 5.1 Expenditure per Thousand on Health, Eastbourne County Borough, 1922/3–36/7
Source: Local Government Financial statistics, 1922/3–1936/7

Politically speaking, Eastbourne was selected as a case study to illustrate a borough with low levels of Labour Party representation. Before 1923 it had no Labour councillors at all. In that year three were elected, and after this date Labour generally held around 10 to 15 per cent of the seats for the rest of the period, and never exceeded 20 per cent.[7] This was considerably below the average for the national dataset, which showed a gradual rise from around 25 per cent of seats to around 35 per cent between 1923 and 1930, followed by some fall and recovery.[8] It was also well below some of the other case study boroughs considered here, as was illustrated particularly forcefully for Barnsley. While Labour councillors were vocal on the council in Eastbourne, they were unable to make any real impact on policies and remained marginal to the decision making on the most important com-

7 'The Municipal Election,' *The Eastbourne Chronicle*, 3 January 1923.
8 See Chapter 3, Figure 3.7c.

mittees.[9] This cannot therefore be called upon as a particularly significant influence on high levels of spending on health services, especially since the years of highest relative levels of expenditure were at the start of the interwar period, when Labour representation was at its lowest.

Instead, two other significant factors emerge from our reading of council minutes and other commentaries on the borough's politics and municipal provision. The first was its high rateable property values, which allowed it to spend at a high level without having to worry about setting an unduly high tax burden on its (generally well-off) residents. This was not the case in some of our other case studies, most notably Barnsley and West Hartlepool. The second reason driving high levels of spending in Eastbourne was the depth of civic pride in the town. This comes across repeatedly in the council proceedings and the local paper – *The Eastbourne Chronicle* – and was particularly felt by certain key players with significant influence over policy decisions. In particular, councillors were concerned to maintain the town's status in relation to other rival resorts, and this prompted the expending of considerable energy and resources over the long term on what may be broadly described as environmental health services. Efforts were made, for example, to improve the sea front, expand the provision of public toilets, build a well appointed Turkish baths, tackle the issue of dog fouling and generally to ensure that the streets were kept clean and pleasant. On one occasion, when challenged by middle-class ratepayers over an increase in the level of rates, the Mayor pointed out that along with keeping the rates down, the council's other duty was 'to up the character of Eastbourne as a high class watering place ... If the reputation

9 See for example 'Town Council,' *The Eastbourne Chronicle*, 6 February 1926; 'Town Council Meeting,' *The Eastbourne Chronicle*, 11 May 1929. In 1937 the Labour group had eight councillors, and demanded to have representation on the Finance Committee, arguing that that whereas Devonshire Ward was to have four representatives on that committee, Roselands and Old Town had none, meaning a 'third of the ratepayers were to go unrepresented on the Council's most important Committee.' They lost this argument, but gained representation on the Entertainments Committee. See 'Labour and Council Committees,' *The Eastbourne Chronicle*, 13 November 1937.

of the town went down, the general prosperity of the place would suffer.'[10] We see this also in a commitment to flagship institutions for health care, like the infectious disease and TB hospitals, and also the voluntary institution, the Princess Alice.

There was another significant factor behind this prioritising of environmental health issues and hospital building, and this was the person of Dr William Willoughby, the MOH. If wealth and civic pride set out the main concerns of Eastbourne's council, Willoughby was instrumental in shaping the form that they took in terms of policy decisions. He was a long-serving and loyal officer, whose medical preferences often reflected his late nineteenth-century training. It will be shown that much of Eastbourne's overall policy on municipal health matters had a conservative shine as a result; part of a legacy from the period of pernicious infectious disease towards the end of the nineteenth century. Nonetheless, Willoughby was a significant force for action, unlike the long-serving MOH in Newport. The remainder of this chapter will focus on these three key factors in explaining Eastbourne's expenditure on health services. The discussion will indicate how far a strong-minded individual could shape policy, regardless of political colour – but also how far this was facilitated by a background level of local affluence.

The Influence of Dr William Willoughby

Willoughby became MOH in Eastbourne in 1894 and remained in post until his retirement in 1939. His tenure thus lent a considerable degree of continuity to local health policies, but also explains an ongoing commitment to what can be termed old fashioned forms of health care in a more modern age. His emphasis on sanitary improvements had raised

10 'Town Council: The Rates: Middle Class Protest', *The Eastbourne Chronicle*, 12 March 1921.

the reputation of the borough in his early years in office: his obituary in the *British Medical Journal* in 1949 stated that under his management it 'became from a sanitary point of view one of the most progressive places in the kingdom'.[11] Willoughby remained committed to his pet methods throughout his career, for example, preferring isolation and home visits to using X-rays in the diagnosis of TB, and rejecting the use of a new serum to treat scarlet fever.[12] His influence was large across the local health services: he was not only the MOH but also the School Medical Officer, both clinical and administrative TB Officer, and the Medical Officer of the infectious diseases hospital. In this latter capacity he visited the hospital every day and supervised the treatment of patients. Compared to many other Medical Officers of Health, Willoughby's clinical and administrative workload was significant, as was his personal control over municipal health policies and priorities.

Willoughby ran a tight ship on the council. He had a good working relationship with local medical practitioners and unusually for a MOH, also achieved a high profile nationally. Both of these achievements were recognised by the Ministry of Health inspectors in 1935, who described him as

> [One] of the most experienced and capable MOH[s] in the country. He is a very good administrator, and a sound clinician. He personally does a good deal of work which many MOH[s] delegate to subordinates ... he takes a broad view of his duties, and endeavours to coordinate all the medical services of the County Borough. He is persona grata with the medical profession in town, and his relations with the voluntary hospitals are excellent.[13]

11 'Obituary: W. G. Willoughby, MD DPH', *British Medical Journal*, 20 August 1949, p. 442.

12 The MOH in Barnsley was using this to good effect by the 1930s (TNA MH66/1066, Survey Report, Barnsley, 46 & 49).

13 TNA MH66/1071, Survey Report, Eastbourne, 7. See also A. M. Lester, 'William George Willoughby, MD, DPH, Medical Officer of Health to Eastbourne, 1894–1939', *Eastbourne Medical Gazette*, 3:1 (1983), who describes Willoughby as 'a great raconteur with a marked sense of humour and a fund of stories'.

In 1931 he became President of the BMA (the first full-time MOH to hold this position) and had a permanent place on the BMA's Public Health Committee.[14] He was also President of the Society of Medical Officers and of the Medical Officers of Schools Association. *The Medical Officer*, the mouthpiece of the Society of Medical Officers, regularly printed extracts of his annual reports, noting that what 'he presents is of more than local value and we shall not forget it'.[15] Willoughby was thus clearly a much respected clinician and administrator, both in Eastbourne and further afield.

This high regard led to a habitual (though not automatic, as we will see) deferral to his suggestions by council committees. Willoughby used his reports to council to suggest changes to provision, where other Medical Officers of Health simply listed birth, death and infectious disease rates.[16] Council minutes suggest strongly that his recommendations were passed with little debate, although this was to change towards the end of the inter-war period. Nonetheless, this relationship between the Medical Officer and council was unusually easy and congenial; it contrasts markedly with that of most of his peers nationally. Willoughby had a much greater impact on the direction of the health services than any of the MOHs in our other case studies. The extent and force of his influence created a well directed service, but it was one that was peppered with certain idiosyncrasies. For example, he did much of his business with local doctors via informal contacts which are largely invisible in the records. This is only revealed in the Ministry of Health survey of the town, where the inspectors observed that although there were few formal consultations between Willoughby and the town's doctors over TB patients, cooperation was 'closer and more constant than the figures would suggest.' This was because of his 'constant and cordial' contact with local practitioners, and the fact that he was 'always "on duty", even on private or social occasions'.[17] A second idiosyncrasy was his already noted reluctance to embrace new techniques such as X-rays.

14 TNA MH66/1071, Survey Report, Eastbourne, 7–8.

15 'The Health of Eastbourne', *The Medical Officer*, vol.38, 3 December 1927, p. 247.

16 Contrast this, for example, with the minutes of Barnsley's Public Health Committee. See Chapter four.

17 TNA MH66/1071, Survey Report, Eastbourne, Survey of the Tuberculosis and Orthopaedic Services.

Willoughby's preferences undoubtedly oiled the machinery of the health services in the town in some ways, but in other respects he held back its progress. The Ministry of Health inspector suggested that he was 'probably not as ready to adopt recent methods as a younger man may be', and his aversion to the use of X-ray to diagnose TB resulted in local doctors bypassing the municipal TB dispensary in early or doubtful cases, and instead sending these patients straight to the TB hospital.[18] The Ministry inspector also noted that the infectious disease hospital (which otherwise attracted favourable notice) could be 'more economically worked' with a cubicle ward system.[19] Willoughby, however, favoured greater isolation, even when there were not enough patients to fill one block.

Willoughby was not alone in his conservative approach to the health services. Many of the other members of the Public Health and related committees were also long-serving, which promoted a general attachment to existing policies. The Assistant MOH, Dr Coghill, for example, was in post for almost as long as Willoughby, and policies were pursued over long periods of time without change. This was enhanced by generally convivial and social relations between council members, producing what might be termed a 'cosy consensus' in health debates and policies in Eastbourne for much of our period.

The last years of the 1930s do however, present a different picture. Although we cannot quantify the change in expenditure on the health services owing to the absence of Local Government Financial Returns after 1936/7, evidence from the council's committees suggest that there was a downturn in spending in the borough after this date. Councillors and other municipal officials also became increasingly combative when presented with Willoughby's proposals, generally on the grounds of cost and the need for economy. The later 1930s saw challenges to improvements to the PAI (the ex Poor Law infirmary), St Mary's, and the extension of the maternity home, and a general move to reduce expenditure. Perhaps more significantly was the change in outlook by the end of our period, which

18 TNA MH66/1071, Survey Report, Eastbourne, Survey of the Tuberculosis and Orthopaedic Services.

19 Ibid. 21.

equated expenditure with wastefulness rather than improved services. As the Borough Treasurer observed over the town's budget for 1938–9:

> It is very difficult to understand why it should be necessary for Eastbourne to expend so much more than Bournemouth and Hastings on Public Assistance, Police, Education and Public Health, for no doubt the services are administered efficiently in those towns, although probably not as elaborately.[20]

The comparison with other resort towns on the south coast is revealing of Eastbourne's constant eye to its public image, but here it is used to justify lowering expenditure. The choice of the term 'elaborate' is also key to understanding the borough's attitude to and pride in its municipal health service for much of this period. The following sections will discuss two of the principal characteristics of this comprehensive, but ultimately economising service: the focus on hospitals, and the relationship with the voluntary sector. Both go a long way to explain the form of Eastbourne's municipal health provision.

The Hospital Ideal in Eastbourne

The commitment to the development of institutions for the delivery of health care is demonstrated in a number of different areas. The infectious disease schemes, for example, heavily favoured the sixty-two-bed isolation hospital (Downside) even where this resulted in poor economies of scale. The council's spending levels on Downside were among the highest in the country in terms of patient costs per week, partly because of low patient numbers. In 1922 a committee found that there were three times as many staff as patients, but this was supported on the grounds that it was insurance against an epidemic: '[c]onsidering the reputation of Eastbourne as a health

20 ESRO DE/A5/12, Eastbourne Finance and General Purposes Committee Minutes, 23 February 1938.

resort the Committee feel that it is money well spent.'[21] The 1933 Ministry of Health survey singled out the infectious disease hospital for praise in helping to maintain a low level of disease in the borough; a situation assisted by generally good housing, low unemployment and a favourable climate. The inspector also noted how far Willoughby was personally involved in supervising the isolation of patients and visiting contacts promptly.[22] He was, however, vocal in vetoing a plan mooted in 1935 to entitle East Sussex County Council to use beds at Downside, indicating how far he was concerned with ring-fencing facilities for his own borough. This portrays Willoughby in an unusually parochial light given his wider involvement in medical societies.[23] The ongoing emphasis on the infectious disease hospital also stands in contrast with our other case studies, although the problems of dealing with other users were more common.

The MCW services were also particularly focused on the maternity home rather than the drop-in and outpatient clinics and milk schemes, as elsewhere. These had developed promptly in Eastbourne: its first Health Visitor was appointed in 1909, and a MCW clinic was opened in 1915.[24] The immediate aftermath of the war saw further vigorous activity on the

21 'Municipal Economy Inquiry' *The Eastbourne Chronicle*, 20 January 1923.

22 TNA MH66/1071, Survey Report, Eastbourne, 15–17. In the case of diphtheria the antitoxin was provided free of charge, but the patient was expected to pay if they were able to afford to do so.

23 ESRO DE/A7/10, Eastbourne Sanitary and Public Health Committee Minutes, Hospitals and Tuberculosis Sub-Committee Minutes, 18 February 1935. Ultimately it was agreed that Eastbourne would build a new cubicle block reserved for cases of certain specified diseases from Hailsham Rural District Council only. Hailsham was to pay the loan charges, a maintenance charge, and a mileage fee for the new ambulance. In fact, as Willoughby later acknowledged, there was ample provision for both Eastbourne and the surrounding authorities at Downside (ESRO DE/A7/8, Eastbourne Sanitary and Public Health Committee minutes, 18 March 1935). It may be significant that Willoughby was allowed three months' sick leave very shortly after this, needing 'complete rest'. His contradictory stance on the usership of the hospital might thus reflect a period of stress which affected his judgement.

24 H. W. Fovargue, *Municipal Eastbourne, 1883–1933 – Selections From the Proceedings of the Town Council* (Eastbourne, 1933), Appendix on health services written by Dr Willoughby, 142.

part initially of the Sanitary and then the MCW Committee, and the council was prompt in adopting the comprehensive MCW scheme proposed by Willoughby in 1918. This included a new municipal maternity home, Upperton House, which became the heart of the service.[25] By 1930, 46 per cent of the borough's births were taking place under the auspices of the maternity home, indicating its popularity.[26] In addition to the municipal home at Upperton House, maternity beds were also provided at the voluntary Bell Hostel for Unmarried Mothers and the poor law infirmary, and further provision was available at the general voluntary hospital, the Princess Alice.

While investment in the MCW schemes remained significantly above average right up to 1936, however, the later 1930s saw a creeping economising compared with the earlier period, and this affected further investment in the maternity home. This reflects the growing tendency towards economy mentioned already, and also illustrates the waning of Willoughby's star towards the end of his period in office. The 1920s saw a series of extensions to the home even when this involved substantial costs, and also its approval as a training home for midwives. This outlook was based on a strong commitment to the need for a good service: in 1920 the Chair of the Sanitary Committee, Councillor Hollins, had justified a considerable overspend on the initial conversion of Upperton House on the grounds of quality, reportedly stating that '[t]he amount spent had been well spent in enabling Eastbourne to have one of the best equipped child welfare centres in the country.'[27] In 1925 Willoughby called the antenatal service one of the 'most

25 It also included clinics shared with the School Medical Services, and free and reduced-cost milk schemes for new and expectant mothers. There was also a municipal midwife and a home help (ESRO DE/A7/8, Eastbourne Sanitary and Public Health Committee Minutes, Report of Maternity and Child Welfare Meeting Held 16 December 1918.

26 TNA MH66/1071, Survey Report, Eastbourne, 26.

27 'Town Council,' *The Eastbourne Chronicle*, 9 October 1920. The overspend was by £340.4.8d (ESRO DE/A7/8, Eastbourne Sanitary and Public Health Committee Minutes, 16 August, 1920). On the training of midwives see ESRO DE/A7/13, Eastbourne Maternity and Child Welfare Committee Minutes, 18 September, 1922.

conspicuous advances' in MCW work in the borough, and along with the health visitor service, 'the backbone to successful work'.[28] The Ministry of Health survey of the borough's health services in 1933 judged that 'on the whole the standard of antenatal work in Eastbourne is good ... The Home is well conducted and very popular.'[29] By 1935, however, plans for further extensions (although ultimately approved) attracted much greater opposition on the grounds of high costs compared with similar homes elsewhere.[30] This did have an impact on the quality of the service: a 1937 Ministry of Health inspection flagged up several deficiencies, but rather than prompting expansion, as earlier, it led only to inaction.[31]

28 MOH Annual Report, Eastbourne, 1925, viii.

29 In 1932, 32 women attended the central health clinic for antenatal purposes, while 320 used the maternity home for the same purpose. TNA MH66/1071, Survey Report, Eastbourne, 28–9.

30 Information from the Ministry of Health quoted in the MCW Committee showed that in 1933 the average cost of municipal maternity homes was £4.18s per patient per week, while at Upperton House it was £5.4.2d (ESRO DE/A7/13, Eastbourne Maternity and Child Welfare Committee Minutes, 15 May 1933). Willoughby claimed that the Eastbourne costs included those left out elsewhere, and later calculated the true cost of keeping a patient in the home for a week at £5.15.6d, which was much more in line with the average cost of similar sized municipal maternity homes. Eastbourne Maternity and Child Welfare Committee minutes, 8 February 1937. For the 1935 decision and subsequent hold-ups and discussion see ESRO DE/A7/13, Eastbourne Maternity and Child Welfare Committee Minutes, 16 September 1935, 20 January 1936, 17 February 1936, 9 March 1936, 30 March 1936, 20 April 1936. See also, 'The Proposed Enlargement of the Maternity Home,' *The Eastbourne Chronicle*, 9 May 1936 and 'Maternity Home Extension: An Alderman's Personal Explanation,' *The Eastbourne Chronicle*, 12 February 1938. The delay was because a plan was put forward to extend maternity provision at the transferred institution, St Mary's. See below for more on this institution.

31 One of these deficiencies was a shortage of municipal midwives, although Willoughby himself judged that Eastbourne was already complying with the terms of the 1936 Midwives Act, and its coverage does seem to have been comparable with Barnsley's. ESRO DE/A7/12, Eastbourne Sanitary and Public Health Committee Minutes, 22 November 1937, where a letter from the Ministry of Health was presented on Eastbourne's compliance with the Midwives Act. In early 1939 it was decided to appoint another municipal midwife, but only at the cost of not employing an

The TB services illustrate the same trend towards prioritising institutional over outpatient facilities. Here, the balance of effort – both in terms of expenditure and staff dedication – tipped towards the TB hospital (Gildredge, opened in 1914) rather than the town dispensary.[32] For example, in 1920 the TB Consultative Sub-Committee reported that it had overshot its estimates for the last seven months by £1,184.18.1d, and that this was mainly through extra expenditure on the institutional treatment of TB (by £775.8.10), and extra costs at Gildredge (of £392.1.11d).[33] This shows the willingness to fund this aspect of the service at least up to 1930, although there were also inefficiencies at work which were later reined in. In the second half of our period, however, expenditure on TB services fell relative to national investment, and also in absolute terms, as is illustrated in Figure 5.2. Patient costs remained above the borough average throughout the period, but were cut significantly from their height of £3 10. 0d per capita per week in 1929 to closer to £2, largely by cutting back on what was seen as extravagant non-essentials.[34] This pattern contrasts with the trend in MCW services, where plans for expansion were increasingly challenged, but where this did not actually translate into cuts being made.

---

additional health visitor (ESRO DE/A7/12, Eastbourne Sanitary and Public Health Committee Minutes, 23 January and 13 February 1939).

32 Clarke, *History of the Eastbourne Medical Society*, Appendix 4. Gildredge was close to the isolation hospital, had good links with the voluntary hospitals of the town and took both council-funded and fee-paying private patients (the former paid according to means). It held twenty four beds for advanced cases. On fees see ESRO DE/A7/8, Eastbourne Sanitary and Public Health Committee Minutes, 16 October 1922.

33 ESRO DE/A7/8, Eastbourne Sanitary and Public Health Committee Minutes, 20 December 1920. Eastbourne sent its sanatorium cases to Nayland and Papworth and children were sent to Wyton Sanatorium: 'In other cases we have to take our chance.' MOH Annual Report, Eastbourne, 1920, p. 50. Other schemes for expansion in the 1920s were, however, turned down on the grounds of expense (see ESRO DE/A7/8, Eastbourne Sanitary and Public Health Committee Minutes, Sanatorium and Baths Sub-Committee Minutes, 10 January 1921, and the annual reports of the MOH).

34 The health committee noted in 1933 that Gildredge was ranked fifth highest on a list of spending costs per capita for similar-sized hospitals (the average cost per patient per week was £2.10.8d compared with Gildredge's £2.11.3d). Enquiries were ordered to be made into further cost cutting, for example, in the gardening staff. Eastbourne Hospitals and Tuberculosis Committee minutes, 22 May 1933.

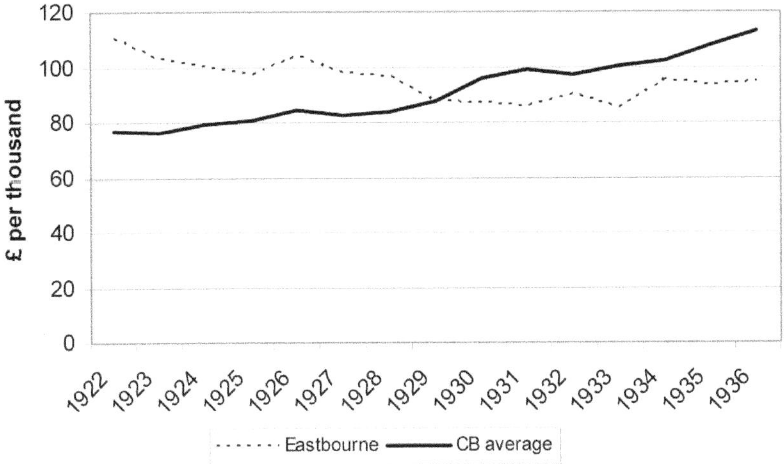

Figure 5.2 Expenditure on TB Schemes, Eastbourne, 1922/3–36/7
Source: Local Government Financial statistics, 1922/3–36/7

Although Willoughby was instrumental in shaping the TB service, his own particular commitment was to the work done at the outpatient dispensary, where he was the Chief TB Officer (unusually for a County Borough MOH, who would generally be simply the administrative Medical Officer). Two clinics were run every week at the Town Hall, one each for men and women, and a special clinic was also run for child patients.[35] Close links were maintained with the various institutions, but Willoughby's reluctance to adopt newer diagnostic and treatment tools like X-rays meant that the dispensary was left behind, and standards there fell.[36] The Ministry of Health inspector in 1933 found several deficiencies in the dispensary's medical services, some of which were based on the failure to adopt modern techniques.[37] Overall, the evidence suggests that the standard of treatment

35 MOH Annual Report, Eastbourne, 1921, p. 53.
36 Willoughby apparently used X-rays only five times in 1931, and once in 1932. TNA MH66/1071, Survey Report, Eastbourne, 71.
37 TNA MH66/1071, Survey Report, Eastbourne, letter from Ministry of Health to Town Clerk, Eastbourne, 22 December 1933.

and care outside the TB hospital was patchy and underused; a fact of which Willoughby seems not to have been aware.[38] The inspector's criticisms did lead to a somewhat increased use of X-rays at the dispensary in the early 1930s and greater efforts to trace contacts, but Willoughby stated that it was an uphill struggle to enforce attendance.[39] In 1935 the dispensary moved to improved accommodation in a new (long-postponed) multi-purpose clinic, Avenue House, but this does not seem to have led to an increase in attendances.[40]

The shape of the TB services joins the picture of the MCW (and also the schemes for VD) to underline again the general commitment to institutional facilities in Eastbourne, and also the changed attitude to expenditure generally by the later 1930s. This was voiced in the context of many of the proposed schemes, but had particular effect for the TB hospital and, to a lesser extent, for the council's maternity home. Spending decisions were, however, also affected by the plans for a unified health scheme, and the place of the transferred PAI in particular. The final section of this chapter will address this topic, which is also instrumental to our understanding of the form of the borough's health service in this period.

38 Attendance was even lower than in West Hartlepool, where we know the dispensary was ill-equipped and unattractive (see Chapter 7). The voluntary sector was represented by the Eastbourne Voluntary Care Committee.

39 TNA MH66/596, Survey Report Correspondence, Eastbourne, Minute by Dr Candler, 12 September 1934. While Willoughby was using X-rays to a greater extent, they were still not being used in conjunction with artificial pneumo-thorax, which was another clinical method the inspector felt was being under-used. Nonetheless, by 1937 and 1938 Willoughby was ordering 58 and 40 X-rays respectively, and the number of sputum samples taken from patients had also risen. MOH Annual Reports, Eastbourne, 1933, pp. 86–7; 1937, p. 91; 1938, p. 111.

40 These stood at 7.3 attendances per case per year when the survey was conducted in 1933, and 7.9 in 1937, after the dispensary had moved to its new premises Figures are from the MOH Annual Reports (unfortunately these are missing for the years 1934–6). Willoughby had repeatedly complained about the conditions and volume of work of some of his staff in the years prior to the move to the new health centre, and this also had an adverse impact on several of the clinics, especially those for VD (ESRO DE/A7/8, Eastbourne Sanitary and Public Health Committee Minutes, 22 January and 19 February 1934). The new clinic had been held up for reasons of economy.

The Question of Appropriation and the Creation of a Unified Health Service in Eastbourne

At the passing of the 1929 Local Government Act Eastbourne County Borough inherited St Mary's PAI from the Poor Law Guardians. It was located in the old town, and although built to house one hundred and twenty patients, by 1933 it had a total of 185 beds.[41] By the early 1930s it consisted of two hospital blocks: an older one built in 1892 and a more modern one completed in 1928, which also housed a nursery for healthy children. The hospital parts comprised a nurses' block, a maternity block, shelters for TB patients and an X-ray/physiotherapy department (although the X-ray equipment was obsolete) which included a masseur. The Ministry inspector in 1933 described the wards as 'well constructed and reasonably well designed, and suitable for first class hospital work. They are well lighted, ventilated and heated. The annexes are modern and satisfactory'.[42] In addition there was a modern operating unit, again seen by the Ministry as well equipped and containing good natural light, although the operating lamp was 'poor'. One of the main concerns of the inspector was the non-classification of patients. There were some separate ward blocks, for children and some chronic patients, but in general 'medical, surgical, acutely ill and chronically ill patients are mixed together in the rest of the Institution'.[43]

The medical staff were likewise judged to be doing high quality work within certain limits. The hospital had only one Medical Officer, who was part-time and not resident, but was a 'good class general practitioner'. There was also one consulting surgeon, a radiologist, a pathologist, Dr Shera (also the council's VD officer), an orthopaedic surgeon, an ophthalmologist, and a dental surgeon. The breadth of work covered by these officers meant that the surgical work was 'of a better standard' than the medical work, except

41 Clarke, *History of the Eastbourne Medical Society*, Appendix 4.

42 TNA MH66/1071, Survey Report, Eastbourne, 48–9.

43 Ibid. 49–50.

for the surgery of bones and joints which was 'less modern than average', but was nevertheless still 'adequate'.[44] Willoughby also led a campaign to have the hospital granted recognition as a full training school for nurses in order to attract more permanent nursing staff, and thus reduce the costs of hiring agency cover.[45] The Ministry initially expressed some concern over the measure 'because the amount of clinical material is decidedly limited, and in spite of some increase in the number of acutely ill surgical patients, the amount of operative surgery is small'.[46] However, the scheme was continued after a probationary year, and it led to considerable economies in the staffing costs.[47] The hospital thus had a range of services already in place at its transfer to the County Borough, with some limitations, and early on showed the potential for improvement while economising on costs (here, of staffing). Further improvements, however, rapidly became bound up with debates about the wider plans for the hospital and its function within the borough's health service.

The option of appropriating St Mary's was not seriously pursued at this stage; in fact although it clearly contained some excellent facilities, the Ministry of Health did not push it, largely because of its cramped town-centre site. The council concurred, and the declarations it made on the future of the institution did not include an intention of formal

44 Ibid. 51–2; Wellcome Institute for the History of Medicine, BMA SA/BMA/F.93, Public Health Files, Contemporary Medical Archives Centre: Completed Questionnaires and Correspondence with Local Authorities and County Boroughs, 1934–5, Eastbourne, returned 1 February 1935. A resident House Surgeon was appointed in 1935, and two full-time consulting surgeons (ESRO R/C50/4, St Mary's Institution and Hospital Sub-Committee, House Sub-Committee Minutes, 19 January 1935).

45 ESRO R/C50/4, House Sub-Committee minutes, 11 October 1932 and 16 March 1933; ESRO DE/A5/9, Finance and General Purposes Committee minutes, 12 June 1933, 10 July 1933.

46 TNA MH66/1071, Survey Report, Eastbourne, 52. See also 'Council Approve New Band Contract', *The Eastbourne Chronicle*, 10 June 1933.

47 ESRO R/C50/4, House Sub-Committee Minutes, 13 March 1934. Numbers of nurses were increased with the opening of a new ward and the conversion of another in 1934.

appropriation.[48] The Public Assistance Committee – largely ex-Guardians, and proud of their institution – were still committed to improvement, however, and of removing any residual poor law stigma attached to its use.[49] Certain councillors were not convinced by this aim, feeling that without appropriation, the PAC was trying to raise St Mary's above its station and to compete with the town's voluntary hospitals. Early on, therefore, St Mary's was placed in a position where it was felt by some that it should not try to emulate the voluntary institutions, while already carrying out some acute and surgical work.

This tension was exacerbated by continued improvements at the PAI which tended it towards the remit of a general hospital: wards were rearranged to increase bed numbers, and new regimes were offered, including radium treatment.[50] Its usership increased, and a greater range of acute treatments were carried out.[51] The Ministry inspector in 1933 judged that since the council had taken over St Mary's the amount of hospital work had

48 The council were advised by the Ministry of Health that they could not reserve beds for patients admitted under the Public Health Acts without appropriation – although in other boroughs (including Newport) this was done. TNA MH66/595, Survey Report Appendices, Eastbourne, Appendix O.

49 The PAC was characterised in these terms by the Town Clerk in 1934 in a report on appropriation. ESRO DE/A7/8, Eastbourne Sanitary and Public Health Committee Minutes, 17 December 1934.

50 ESRO R/C50/4, House Sub-Committee Minutes, 12 May 1931, 21 November 1933. See also 'Should St Mary's be a General Hospital?', *The Eastbourne Chronicle*, 8 December 1934.

51 ESRO R/C50/4, House Sub-Committee Minutes, 16 March 1933. The average number of beds filled in 1932 was 154.8, while for 1931 it was 148. For the first part of 1933 the average was 181, and for the corresponding quarter of the previous year it was 165. See also BMA SA/BMA/F.93, Contemporary Medical Archives Centre: Completed Questionnaires and Correspondence with Local Authorities and County Boroughs, 1934–5, Eastbourne. BMA Public Health files, Completed Questionnaire, Eastbourne. There was also some support from the Borough Treasurer and the Finance and PACs for developing the town's municipal maternity service at St Mary's, although ultimately Upperton House was favoured (as Willoughby and the Sanitary Committee had hoped). For the debates on the motion see ESRO DE/A5/12, Eastbourne Finance and General Purposes Committee minutes, 27

increased 'both in volume and in the proportion of cases needing active medical or surgical treatment.' The uneasy position relative to the voluntary hospitals was also being improved via the establishment of a Joint Hospital Committee to facilitate co-operation between the two sectors. As a result 'some measure of interchange of patients has been established.'[52] At this stage Willoughby supported the appropriation of St Mary's, stating that it would facilitate cooperation with the voluntary hospitals, particularly the Princess Alice, which largely treated surgical cases and did not like keeping patients for long periods of time. St Mary's could therefore develop its role as a general hospital serving long-staying patients.[53] He did not press his opinion particularly forcefully, however, concluding rather insipidly in 1935 that 'if it does not cost much it would be a nice thing to do.'[54]

Willoughby's view was underpinned by an inclination to see voluntary and municipal hospital facilities as part of one whole. In a 1930 survey of hospital accommodation of his own, he judged that taken together 'the present accommodation at the combined hospitals is probably just sufficient for the present needs of the Borough as regards adults ...', although that for children was deficient.[55] The Ministry inspector in 1933 was of a similar opinion albeit without supporting appropriation. He recommended improvements at St Mary's, the amalgamation of the four voluntary hospitals and the co-ordination of services between the two sectors.[56] Indeed, his report stated that the existence of a PAI alongside four separate voluntary hospitals in a town the size of Eastbourne was 'regrettable'.[57] Both the Ministry inspector and Willoughby thus supported co-ordination and

---

September 1936 and 'Costly Improvement Schemes,' *The Eastbourne Chronicle*, 10 October 1936.

52 TNA MH66/1071, Survey Report, Eastbourne, letter from Ministry of Health to Town Clerk, Eastbourne, 22 December 1933.

53 Ibid. 54–5.

54 Ibid. Correspondence, note of interview between Eastbourne County Borough delegates and Ministry of Health, 13 February 1935.

55 MOH Annual Report, Eastbourne, 1938, pp. 30 & 32.

56 TNA MH66/1071, Survey Report, Eastbourne, p. 66.

57 Ibid. 60.

specialisation within one overall hospital service, although their opinions on appropriation differed. By 1939, however, St Mary's had been improved to the extent that the Ministry was now also urging appropriation.[58]

This situation serves to illustrate the variety of courses a borough could pursue after 1929, and the ways that these interacted specifically with local conditions. Eastbourne had enviably good medical facilities at its PAI, but its existing reputation was such that appropriation was not felt to be necessary outside PAI and MOH circles. In this case, it was the Finance Committee and the Borough Treasurer who particularly opposed it on the grounds that it would bring increased costs, unlike the situation in other boroughs, where the Public Assistance Committee often formed the main opposition.[59] The opponents of appropriation saw the voluntary hospitals as the principal providers of hospital care in the town, and St Mary's as the most junior partner in the overall plan. This reflects Eastbourne's attachment to charitable and self-help rather than rate-supported schemes; a scenario we find also in Newport, although there the municipal schemes were neglected as a result. In Eastbourne the good quality of the PAI raised its profile, as did a section of the council who saw the potential for its continued development.

Nonetheless, as in Newport, there was a tradition of council participation in collaborative schemes with the voluntary sector – as had long been common under the Poor Law Medical Services. The council had user arrangements with all of the voluntary hospitals in some form: it contributed an annual subscription to the Princess Alice in exchange for an informal agreement that it could admit municipal cases, it took voluntary sector probationer nurses at the isolation hospital for six months of their training,

58 ESRO DE/A7/10, Eastbourne Sanitary and Public Health Committee Minutes, Letter from Ministry of Health to Eastbourne County Borough Council, 3 March 1939 recorded in the Minutes for 20 March 1939. This support was strengthened by the institution's recognition as a training school for nurses (see above) and by the fact that it had been recognised under the 1930 Public Assistance Order as an institution concerned solely with the sick.

59 The fear of increased costs on appropriation was a common one, although the Ministry of Health was at pains to state that it was unfounded.

and it gave unspecified donations to the other hospitals for the admission of council patients.[60] This was further smoothed by a close relationship between Willoughby and the voluntary hospital medical officers, and also by the fact that many councillors were members of the respective hospital committees. This commonality of outlook echoes the support from all sides for the voluntary hospital in Barnsley, although in Eastbourne it was at a more elite level of society. It also underlines how much local business was facilitated (or retarded) by face-to-face and personal contacts.

The desire for a unified hospital service (which included St Mary's as a junior partner) was ultimately stymied by poor relations from within the voluntary sector, especially in the early 1930s, rather than between voluntary and municipal bodies.[61] By the later 1930s relations between the Princess Alice and St Mary's had improved, thanks to Willoughby's efforts to triage patients according to need – although this did lead to its own problems over patient charges.[62] This is also the one area where political colour may have played a part in the shaping of Eastbourne's health services, albeit indirectly: appropriation was seen as a political, and specifically Labour, move by some councils, and this may have been a further point against

60 ESRO DE/A7/8, Eastbourne Sanitary and Public Health Committee Minutes, Report of meeting of the Sanatorium Sub-Committee, 15 September, 1919. The arrangement with the ENT hospital ended in 1934 in favour of the council paying for specific cases. ESRO DE/A5/12, Finance and General Purposes Committee Minutes, 26 March 1934. See also J. Surtees, *The Princess Alice and other Eastbourne Hospitals* (Eastbourne, 1994). The London Homeopathic Hospital Convalescent Unit was also sited in Eastbourne, seeing two hundred cases a year. See Clarke, *History of the Eastbourne Medical Society*, Appendix 4. Many of the patients at all these hospitals were from outside Eastbourne.

61 The chair of the Princess Alice Hospital was willing to amalgamate with the ENT hospital, for example, but not with the other hospitals. TNA MH66/1071, Survey Report, Eastbourne, 60–1.

62 This was particularly when patients from the voluntary hospital were moved to St Mary's for treatment. 'Proposed Increased Grant to Princess Alice Hospital', *The Eastbourne Chronicle*, 9 October 1937. Staff at the Princess Alice also complained that the grant they received from the council was insufficient (it was increased in 1937), and staff at St Mary's felt that they were being used as 'a rubbish heap for incurable patients' (TNA MH66/1071, Survey Report, Eastbourne, 61).

it.[63] Ultimately, the position of St Mary's in the wider hospital hierarchy remained ambiguous. It was clearly a good hospital in many respects, but its development was retarded by financial retrenchment and a preference for the voluntary institutions, even after the Ministry of Health started to urge it be appropriated. It did, however, have a working relationship with the primary voluntary hospital by the end of the 1930s, although this was largely informal, and thus prone to confusion. Further coordination within the borough was prevented by an unwillingness to consolidate from within the voluntary sector. While the standard of care available to Eastbourne's residents at its various hospitals was generally high, it was poorly coordinated and planned, largely due to deeply entrenched animosities and feelings about the role of different institutions.

Conclusions

The analysis of Eastbourne's municipal health service has revealed several distinctive characteristics. Those outlined at the start of this chapter were the borough's general affluence, and its civic pride, which allowed it variously to invest at a high level on its services, and gave it the impetus to do so. The character and preferences of the MOH, Dr Willoughby, was a further force in shaping the health services. Willoughby's medical background, plus the council's predisposition towards flagship institutions which would further the borough's reputation for health, led to a focus on the institutional delivery of healthcare in several fields. Over the course of the period, however, these characteristics were joined by an increasingly keen eye to cost-cutting and economy, which led to a loss of the 'cosy consensus' of the earlier period, and a stunting of certain medical schemes.

63 The chairman of the Public Health Committee in Bournemouth told the Ministry inspector in confidence 'that the question [of hospital appropriation] was erroneously regarded as purely political and the overwhelmingly conservative majority looked upon appropriation as a socialist measure which should be opposed' (TNA MH66/476, Survey Correspondence, Bournemouth).

Eastbourne's affluence and general salubriousness not only brought good levels of resources to fund its municipal services, but also low levels of need for certain curative health services compared with many other boroughs (albeit perhaps raised needs associated with its elderly population).[64] We have seen in several cases, however, that this did not preclude councillors from resisting increases in expenditure. They supported an expensive MCW scheme (counter-intuitive given the age profile of the borough), but most of the extensions to the maternity home had to go through a battle to be approved. The TB scheme was subject to a considerable economy drive because of concerns over spending, and the Finance Committee in particular, was intransigent when it came to the more comprehensive plans to improve St Mary's PAI. This latter point relates also to wider feelings about the place of the PAI in the hospital hierarchy, but it demonstrates that economy in the 1930s affected even this affluent borough. In his acceptance speech as Mayor in 1930, Lt.-Col. Gwynne stressed the 'importance of exercising rigid economy ... in these days when money was very tight.'[65]

Despite this economy drive, standards of care continued to be broadly praised by the Ministry of Health. Their involvement did not prevent anomalies in the service, however, the most notable of which was the treatment of St Mary's transferred institution. The Public Assistance Committee led initiatives to improve it, and Ministry of Health assessments were that its services were patchy but generally good. Appropriation was not generally approved of, however, and Willoughby (unusually for a MOH) did not push this particularly. The desire to retain St Mary's as a PAI rather than a public health hospital stemmed largely from the Finance Committee who were averse either to increased costs, or to challenging the supremacy of the voluntary hospitals. In common with Newport, this points to a willingness to view council provision as part of an overall borough service, even when

64 It is also illustrated in the low numbers of Medical Officers (there was only one Assistant MO to work alongside Willoughby, and the Medical Officers for the TB and VD services were part time) and health visitors compared with hospital nursing staff. This produced low reported wage bills for the borough since the latter were not included in the Annual Financial Returns.

65 'Lt.-Col. Gwynne Re-Elected', *The Eastbourne Chronicle*, 15 November 1930.

this down weighted the municipal sector. However it also led to a lack of agreement over the way that St Mary's should be developed, and was let down by disunity within the voluntary sector, and perhaps a suspicion of Labour politics at play as well.

The high levels of investment in the health services were prompted by a genuine desire to provide high quality services for residents and visitors, but it was not uniform across the board The MCW scheme was particularly prioritised, for example, while the TB hospital suffered significant cutbacks. This relates both to the needs of the borough, and to Willoughby's preferences. By the second half of the period, Willoughby's influence on spending decisions was being increasingly challenged, and the Finance Committee instead took on greater significance. In sum, this discussion has confirmed that Eastbourne was a rich and high spending borough, where the Labour Party had little influence. However, this investment was neither uniformly high across the board, nor consistent over the period. By the second half of our period, indeed, the borough was being outstripped by Barnsley in expenditure terms. There, the active and cohesive Labour Party had been instrumental in pushing the development of the health services. In Eastbourne party politics had little role to play; instead it was individuals on the council and long-held attitudes towards different providers and institutions which directed the shape of the municipal services.

CHAPTER SIX

Newport

Newport in Monmouthshire, was an unusual town for a Welsh County Borough – in fact, it can be regarded as the most 'English' of the County Boroughs in Wales, of which there were four (Newport, Cardiff, Swansea and Merthyr Tydfil). This is because of the diversity of its economy and its relative wealth, which contrasts in particular with the very poor borough of Merthyr, which was heavily reliant on the coal mining industry. Nonetheless it was, at least for administrative purposes during our period, firmly 'Welsh', and this forms an important backdrop to our analysis of its health services. Specifically, it adds another tier to our exploration of interwar localism, beyond the explanatory factors of wealth, politics and style of local government. Most significantly, from 1922 Newport was under the purview of the Welsh Board of Health rather than directly under the Ministry of Health, and featured in the health surveys of the interwar period that related specifically to Wales.[1] Furthermore, its TB services were locked into wider Welsh provision via the voluntary Welsh National Memorial Association, which delivered TB care in Wales. This had a significant impact on the delivery of this service beyond the inclinations of the individual councils. This chapter will investigate this aspect of localism as another way into explaining how decisions on health care were made locally. We also examine how Newport's particular characteristics affected the nature of the town's Labour Party and how it operated within the borough. As we suggested in Chapter Three, we would expect a Labour council pres-

1 These were the Welsh Consultative Council, Maternal Mortality Enquiry, 1922–5 (see TNA MH96/907), the Report on Maternal Mortality in Wales, 1937, Cmd. 5423, xi, and the Report of the Committee of Inquiry in the Anti-Tuberculosis Service in Wales and Monmouthshire (London, 1939). Newport also figured in comparative data collected by the Ministry of Health on the County Boroughs of Wales on VD up to 1925 (see TNA MH96/1135, Prevalence of Venereal Disease in Wales, 1918–41).

ence to have a positive impact on the provision of municipally provided health care (as was the case in Barnsley). That a high Labour presence did not correlate with high levels of expenditure in Newport offers us a means of further unpacking the complexities of the interwar municipal health services in England and Wales.

Newport grew up around the docks on the River Usk, serving its iron and steel hinterland, and becoming the largest town in Wales by the 1830s. Its location close to the Severn estuary and the English border meant that transport links via the railway east to Bristol and north towards Shrewsbury also became central to the town's economy. By 1918 around 40 per cent of men in the town were employed in this sector.[2] Its economic profile was thus diverse, and it had a relatively high presence of professional and managerial employments.[3] Consequently, unlike much of south Wales, it was not given depressed Special Area status, as its mix of commerce alongside heavy industry allowed it to better ride out the difficulties of the depression. While unemployment in the borough in 1931 was significant – 16.4 per cent of the male working-age population – it was far below West Hartlepool's 29 per cent and also under Barnsley's 17.9 per cent.[4] With an average size of 94,000 inhabitants over the period it was substantially the largest of our four case studies, but its population was also relatively stable, suffering only a slight reduction in the early 1930s.[5]

Newport was also relatively well-off in terms of its rate base; in fact the rateable value per head of its property was almost exactly the County

2 H. Davis, *The History of the Borough of Newport: From Swamp to Super-town* (Newport, 1998), 232.

3 Newport also contained, 'sheet iron rolling mills, nail and rivet works, brattice cloth, Indian rubber and chemical works, engineering works, shipbuilding yards, iron and brass foundries, cast iron pipe manufacturers, dry docks, saw mills, creosoting works, brick and tile makers, lime kilns, flour mills, clothing factories, tobacco and confectionary manufacturers.' See Davis, *The History of the Borough of Newport*, 234. 1931 census figures are from Davies and Morley, *County Borough Elections* i: *Barnsley–Bournemouth*.

4 Davies and. Morley, *County Borough Elections in England and Wales* i: *Barnsley–Bournemouth*.

5 See Chapter 3, Figure 3.7a for comparative population figures for the four case studies.

Borough average throughout the interwar period. It did not have the property wealth of Eastbourne, which was in a league of its own, but its base level of resources was significantly higher than that in either Barnsley or West Hartlepool. This did not translate into a large income for much of the period, however, as the council chose to keep its rates relatively low – somewhat below the national average except for 1927, when it raised its rate in the pound to approximately the mean.[6] In the following year, however, it was reduced again, both in absolute and relative terms. Residents were thus not taxed unduly, but the income from rates was depressed accordingly. This issue of rates was a significant one for the council: after they had managed to make a reduction of 1/10d in the pound in 1930, councillors would apparently 'readily admit to the fact that the town's ratepayers could not afford some projected scheme or other and would cheerfully postpone it until a more propitious time'.[7]

This reluctance to raise levels of income via higher taxation correlated with below-average levels of spending on health up to 1929 (see Figure 6.1). We have already seen that the rise after the Local Government Act actually coincided with a reduction in the rate in the pound, and we will go on to demonstrate that it was linked to one service in particular which was administered at a higher level: the TB schemes. The wider impact of the 1929 Act may also have played a part, for example, through the changed grant scheme, and the transfer of services to the Public Health Committee. We should note, however, that health was not one of the main priorities of this council: they devoted the smallest share of their overall budget to health services of all of our case studies until 1929 (although there was a gradual rise from 1927 onwards), and they only lost their ranking because of a precipitous fall in relative spending on health in West Hartlepool after 1929.[8]

6 See Chapter 3, Figure 3.7b and e. The average rateable value in Newport was 6–7 pounds per head annually, with a gradual rise of the period. The average rate levied was 10.9 shillings in the pound, compared with a borough average of 11.9. (Annual Financial Returns, 1922/3–36/7).

7 Davis, *The History of the Borough of Newport*, 241.

8 Newport spent an average of 5.7 per cent of its rate fund income on health, compared with a national average of 7.1 per cent (excluding expenditure on appropriated

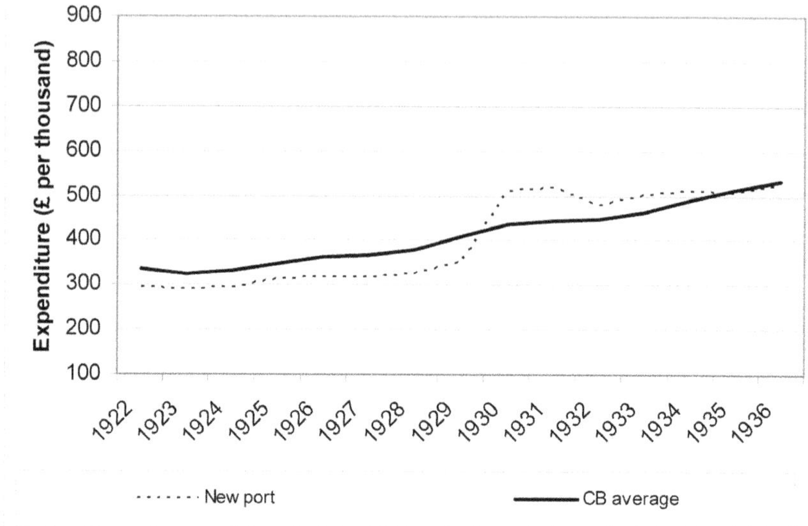

Figure 6.1 Expenditure per Thousand on Health, Newport County Borough, 1922/3–36/7
Source: Local Government Financial statistics, 1922/3–36/7

Indicators of the population's health status are mixed. Having mainly expanded in the late nineteenth century, Newport was 'of comparatively modern growth', with its standard of housing described in the late 1930s as 'on the whole good'.[9] This was in no small measure the result of the council's building programme: it had by 1932 built around three thousand new houses, meaning that levels of overcrowding were relatively low. However in practice a large number of people who required rehousing were unable to afford the rents of the new council homes, resulting in pockets of overcrowding and the development of shanty settlements on the outskirts of the town. Consequently, the 1929 Report of the MOH stated that 'the condi-

hospitals from the national figure as it was not a head addressed by all boroughs – see Chapter 2). Eastbourne was the only one of our case studies to spend at approximately this level over the period as a whole. (Annual Financial Returns, 1922/3–36/7).

9 Report on Maternal Mortality in Wales, 12.

tions under which a large proportion of the poorer people live constitute a serious menace to the health of the community'.[10] By 1939 things seem to have improved, and a TB survey in Wales of that year reported favourably on both the town and its councillors:

> It is very well served ... by an active, energetic and far-seeing Council and officials ... The record of the borough since 1919 is an excellent one. It is their proud claim that Newport has not a slum within its boundaries and indeed has no bad houses, and that overcrowding has almost entirely disappeared. We were greatly impressed by the care and foresight shown in the maintenance of the Council's house property. The council feel justified in saying that they have solved all their housing problems, and that now it is only a question of keeping up their good record from year to year as necessity arises.[11]

The investment in housing may be one reason why the council did not feel so motivated to spend at a high level on the personal health services. This is borne out by the fact that the council had also spent £70,000 over the previous decade improving the sewerage system, and had plans in place to build a reservoir at a cost of £500,000. As a contemporary report put it: '[t]his is indeed a record worthy of note, especially when it is remembered that, in 1935, there were within the borough ten thousand unemployed persons'.[12] This good record in housing was not reflected in its health statistics across the board, however: while its infant mortality rate compared 'very favourably' with the County Borough average, its maternal mortality, pulmonary TB, and other infectious disease rates were consistently higher. In general however, ministry inspectors found that the health services in Newport even in 1932 'on the whole are satisfactory and some very good work is being done'.[13]

10 MOH Annual Report, Newport, 1929, p. 72.

11 Report of the Committee of Inquiry in the Anti-Tuberculosis Service in Wales and Monmouthshire, 186.

12 Ibid., 187.

13 TNA MH96/387, Survey Report, Newport, 4, 7 & 45.

In sharp contrast to West Hartlepool where relations with the Ministry of Health were poor, largely because of the council's reluctance to spend on health schemes (see Chapter Seven), Newport's council managed to keep on good terms with Whitehall and the Welsh Board of Health, while also spending below or around the average on its health services. In part this may have been related to the fact that, as is clear from the above, the council was active in other areas such as housing, which were also under the control of the Ministry of Health. We also find that the micro-study reveals much more than the quantitative figures suggest: not only the emphasis from the council on other services related to health (housing and sewerage), but also the significance of the voluntary sector. Of all our case studies, Newport was the town which relied most heavily on voluntary agencies to fulfil the council's various health service obligations. Unlike the other three towns, it did not have a municipal maternity home, for example, relying initially on a voluntary aided home, and later on, the private sector. We have already noted the significance of the Welsh National Memorial Association in the provision of TB services, and in addition to this the municipal general VD clinic was run by the Royal Gwent Hospital, which was also central to the town's hospital provision. A voluntary committee also ran the infant welfare centres, and the council had furthermore given over its responsibilities under the Blind Acts to a local voluntary committee. This marks Newport out from our other case studies, and will be a central part of our interpretation of the town's priorities for its municipal health services.

It is also crucial to appreciate the role of voluntarism in shaping the role of the Labour Party in the borough. Newport returned a higher than average level of Labour councillors throughout the period (with the exception of 1936), which points to a potential spur for spending on socially ameliorative services, as we saw in Barnsley. Yet the town spent generally less than the average on its health provisions. As we will show below, the local character of the party was crucial both in terms of its (in)ability to gain a foothold in municipal politics and its ability to interact with the other forces – notably voluntary agencies – aiming to improve the health services of the town. The rest of this chapter will attempt to unpick this apparent paradox of a borough with a high Labour presence, but a low level of investment in health. In particular, we will call on the ethos of voluntarism and its role in shaping municipal provision. This could act both in opposition to, as well as in tandem with municipalism (as well as with the Labour Party). While in some cases the reliance on voluntary agencies removed the need for the council to develop its own services, it was not automatically the cheaper choice: using the Welsh National Memorial Association, for example, was in fact an expensive option. Using the workings of the local voluntary blind association as an example, we further amplify our argument that attempting to construct a municipal health service using other agencies could throw up serious issues of governance.

The Low Spending, High Labour Paradox

While Barnsley's Labour Party was dominated by the mining union, Newport's had a very different complexion. Newport had the largest individual membership of the Party in Wales of around two thousand members, and it was amongst the largest parties in Great Britain.[14] This can be contrasted with Barnsley which had roughly 120 individual members in 1928, doubling by 1931 and remaining at a steady level thereafter until 1947.[15] The large membership of the local party meant that Newport was treated as a success story by the national leadership and 'was feted by national leaders and other constituency Labour parties as an organisational model.' Records show that this membership translated into a very visible and socially active party, which by the 1920s was creating its 'own political culture, featuring annual May Day celebrations and a welter of choirs, orchestras, education classes, children's outings and party dances and suppers'. While some activ-

14 D. Tanner, 'The Pattern of Labour Politics, 1918–1939,' in D. Tanner, C. Williams and D. Hopkin, eds, *The Labour Party in Wales, 1900–2000* (Cardiff; 2000), 120–3.

15 T. Lindley, 'The Party Machine: A Study of Barnsley Labour Party and its Leaders, 1918–1945', dissertation for the Social Studies Diploma, Ruskin College, 1978, p. 23.

ities attracted only small numbers, in certain wards Labour clubs drew in a large section of the local population through their social programmes. Alongside this Newport's Labour Party organised a successful and dynamic women's section and, unusually, women were strongly represented on the constituency executive.[16]

Crucially however, with the exception of a short period with a Labour MP, political power was denied at both municipal and parliamentary levels.[17] During the interwar period, despite achieving fifty per cent of councillors in three years, Labour never succeeded in gaining full control. In direct contrast to Barnsley, Newport's Labour Party did not throw up any strong leaders – the admittedly Liberal local newspaper, the *South Wales Weekly Argus* described their leader, Frank Quick as 'inconsistent' and his union refused to allow him to stand for re-election in 1934 in rather murky circumstances.[18] This leadership weakness contributed to the party's inability to seize power without an overall majority. For example, it failed to take the route used in Barnsley of manipulating the aldermanic system in order to gain control.[19] This lack of unity and drive meant that the opportunity to take a majority of seats did not arise again before 1945. A lack of strong leadership, the absence of major unions and the predominance of individual membership seems to have produced a local party in Newport that was strong on social events, but rather weaker when it came to political organisation and impact. This probably further affected their influence over the investment made in health services.

16 D. Tanner, 'Labour and its Membership', in D. Tanner, P. Thane and N. Tiratsoo, eds, *Labour's First* Century (Cambridge, 2000), 251.

17 There are both similarities and differences here with the experience of Preston see M. Savage, 'Rise of the Labour Party in Local Perspective', *Journal of Regional and Local Studies*, 10:1 (1990), 12.

18 'Mr Quick, the "Argus" and Talybont', *South Wales Weekly Argus*, 1 November 1930.

19 An example is the 1934 municipal election result, when Labour took 50 per cent of council seats but was insufficiently united to force through the election of some Labour aldermen. 'Labour to Turn out the Aldermen?', *South Wales Weekly Argus*, 6 October. 1934.

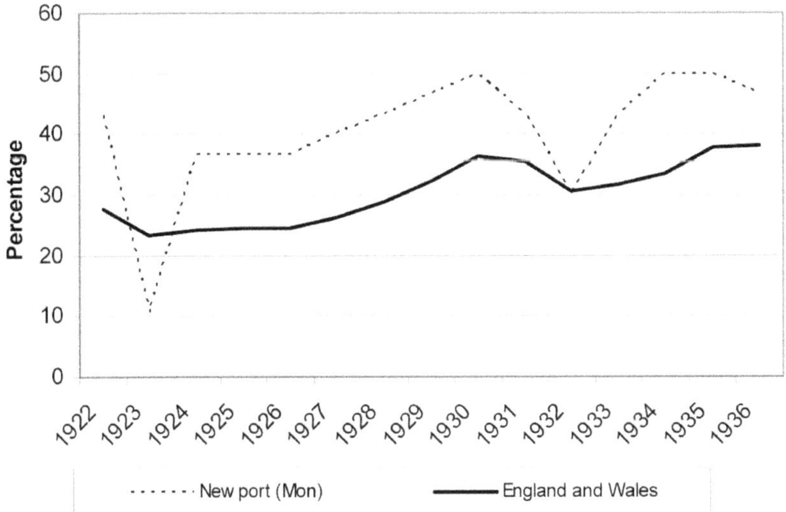

Figure 6.2 Percentage of Labour Seats on Newport council, 1922–36
Source: The *Times* municipal election returns, 1922–36. The returns for 1923 should be treated with caution, as many County Boroughs had apparently anomalous returns.

Although the quantitative side of our project identified Newport as a 'high Labour' local authority, this did not in fact translate into political power for the party at the municipal level. Our analysis of Barnsley and Newport local parties consequently underlines the importance of considering micro-politics as a crucial factor in understanding the development of Labour (and by implication all parties) as a political force. Beyond this, however, are two points that are worth drawing out in the assessment of the provision of health care in the borough. The first is that Labour appeared less interested in the provision of health care than its counterpart in Barnsley; and second, that there was a tradition of relying on the voluntary sector to provide Newport's health service. This again points to the importance of unpicking the role of voluntary services as well as the workings and influences of the council in municipal health care provision.

The lack of political dynamism in the Newport Labour Party compared to that in Barnsley stands in curious contradiction to the assertions of the journal *Searchlight*, the public face of the local Party during election time, and also the minutes of its meetings. Surviving examples of the election publication repeatedly emphasised the commitment to healthcare in particular: that the 'first duty of a council should be to look after the health of the people'.[20] This strategy was very much in line with the broader Labour concerns over women's health in South Wales during the interwar period,[21] and led to election literature (often with an eye to female voters) contrasting current spending on health with that of other services:

> Some facts for Women – the 'business men' of Newport spent £2491 on Maternity and Child Welfare in 1925–6, equal to 1/50 of a penny per head of the town's population; but spent £3356 on the fire brigade, £17,232 on public lighting and £19,997 on the police – This is government by Liberal-Tory businessmen – They think women will allow it to continue. Women! Vote Labour and teach them a lesson.[22]

In addition to election-time literature, there are further suggestions that health was of concern to the local party. Frank Quick, a Labour councillor, was the council representative on the Wales-wide Welsh National Memorial Association, and was a consistent presence on the Health Committee, chairing it in 1928–9. A high profile female local Labour activist, Mrs Lewcock, was likewise prominent on the MCW Committee. Yet while Duncan Tanner agrees with Michael Savage's findings that the large involvement of women resulted in a move away from traditionally male territories, he finds no particular emphasis on MCW specifically or on health more generally in local Labour Party minutes, with the possible exception of the welfare of the blind scheme, which is discussed in more detail below.[23]

20 Newport Reference Library (hereafter NRL), *Searchlight*, 20 October 1923.

21 For further discussion see S. Thompson, 'Unemployment, Poverty and Women's Health in Inter-war Wales', in P. Michael and C. Webster, eds, *Health and Society in Twentieth Century Wales* (Cardiff, 2006), and M. Williams, '"The Growing Toll of Motherhood": Maternal Mortality in Wales', Ibid.

22 'Who are the Spendthrifts?', *The Newport Searchlight*, 1926 municipal election edition.

23 Tanner, 'The Pattern of Labour Politics'; SLA A.1, Records of Newport Constituency Labour Party (hereafter NCLP), Minute Books of the Labour Representation

In fact, whenever MCW was raised, it was typically in relation to a lack of action or progress of the party or of the municipality more generally. Many other local authorities in our wider national study, for example, had established a municipal maternity home by 1922, but it was not until 1935 that a letter from Caerau's Women's Section was passed on to the council Labour Group asking for the provision of a municipal maternity hospital in Newport.[24] And despite the presence of the dynamic Mrs Lewcock, in other areas of MCW the local Labour Party was similarly lacking in initiative. In 1926, following a visit to the Infant Health Central Committee, which coordinated the work of the town, national Party representatives came away 'feeling the need for greater Labour representation in this particular sphere.'[25]

The only health initiative we can definitely attribute to Labour action, and to Quick in particular, was the creation of a new smallpox hospital, located outside the borough boundaries at Crick House. A smallpox epidemic in Newport in the late 1920s highlighted the deficiencies of the increasingly old and substandard isolation facility which, in the words of Quick, was 'not fit for a dying dog'.[26] Using the opportunity of Quick's chairmanship of the Health Committee, and a Labour majority on that committee for the only time in the interwar era, the year 1928–9 saw repeated attempts to find suitable property for such a hospital. Although Crick House was not bought until March 1930, the influence of Quick and his colleagues is made clear in subsequent discussions of the purchase, which were highly politically charged. Crick House was unpopular with neighbouring local authorities and disapproved of by the Ministry of Health on the grounds that it was not, in fact, suitable for smallpox treatment. Perhaps

---

Committee, 18 November and 2 December 1920, 21 March 1921; SLA A.5, Minute Books of the Labour Representation Committee, 13 August and 27 August 1926; SLA A.6, Minute Books of the Labour Representation Committee, 2 May 1930.

24 SLA A.7, NCLP, Minute Books of the Labour Representation Committee, 25 March 1935.

25 SLA A.5, NCLP, Minute Books of the Labour Representation Committee, 12 February 1926.

26 'Condemnation of Cefn Hospital', *South Wales Weekly Argus*, 15 March 1930.

most damningly of all, though, it received in its lifetime not a single smallpox case, the epidemic being over by the time it opened. Quick defended his actions, stating that the council was legally required to provide smallpox accommodation, and that criticism had 'been engineered simply because the Health Committee last year was, to use someone's term, *dominated by a Labour majority'* [emphasis added].[27]

The purchase of Crick House, unfortunate on one level, might nonetheless be seen as an example of a rapid response on the part of a Labour-dominated Health Committee to the twin problems of an aged isolation hospital and a smallpox epidemic. As such, it again clearly illustrates how contingent and highly localised issues were crucial in shaping Labour policy. Taken in the context of Labour's lack of control of the council it also demonstrates how circumscribed its field of opportunity was, and perhaps how limited its drive to improve municipal provision. This latter trend was lent weight, as we show in the next section, by the dominance of voluntary activity in the borough.

The Significance of Voluntarism in Newport

As we have already suggested, the liveliness of the voluntary sector in Newport effectively restricted one of the areas in which Labour was active elsewhere. In this context it is worth noting the relatively high proportion of middle class households in the town mentioned in the introduction. The middle classes were clearly not as dominant as in Eastbourne, but compared to the other County Boroughs of south Wales, they and the locally prominent gentry created a pool of women in particular, able to engage in a range of good works. In this section, we use the examples of the municipality's relationship with the Royal Gwent Hospital and the Welsh National Memorial Association to show how the council relied heavily on

27 'Crick House and Smallpox', *South Wales Weekly Argus*, 13 December 1930.

voluntary organisations to provide its statutory services across a range of areas. While this tendency would appear to spring from the fact that, like Eastbourne, voluntarism had a well-established tradition in the town, we also show how this did not necessarily result in easy or even productive relationships, and sometimes brought greater expense for the council.

Voluntarism provides us with the context for the failure of the party to expand into the arena of MCW, which elsewhere was such a central part of its activities. Labour never gained more than a minor foothold on the local Infant Health Central Committee. This committee was first established in 1908 and was made up of lady volunteers and the members of the council's Health Committee. It was dominated by the great and the good of the area, including in its ranks Viscountess Rhondda and the locally prominent Tredegar family, and was neither overtly political nor radical in its outlook. Thus, unlike other towns such as Barnsley, where the provision of free milk rapidly became tied to a broader principle of municipal socialism, in Newport it was far more closely tied with the tradition of (upper) middle class female voluntary activity.

This voluntary committee was extremely active, particularly in the 1920s, when it played a central role in the provision of services at the infant welfare centres. Volunteers ran sewing and knitting clubs, organised health education and cookery lectures, and provided a crèche service at the centres. Voluntary contributions paid for the interest on savings in the Maternity Clubs and for the supply of flannel for children's clothes at or below cost price, and subsidised fireguards.[28] A major aspect of its work in the infant welfare centres was the provision of free or reduced price milk to necessitous children, in which capacity it acted as a significant supplement to the municipal milk scheme: in the 1920s voluntary spending on this item equalled, or commonly exceeded the amount spent by the council.[29] This was in direct contrast to Barnsley, where the substantial milk programme was an entirely municipal affair.

28 MOH Annual Report, Newport, 1925, p. 20.

29 GCRO A110. M26–37, Maternity and Child Welfare Committee Minutes, Newport County Borough Council General Council minutes, 1920–30.

Significantly, voluntary provision was also vital in establishing maternity care in the town, removing the imperative for the council to provide its own home. A voluntary maternity home had been established in Herbert Street in 1904 in order to 'provide skilled nursing for the wives of the working classes and to train midwives'. By the end of the First World War, it was taking about 500 maternity cases and also training around twenty midwives a year.[30] The council reserved a bed at this home for its cases in return for a fixed annual fee and a weekly charge, and when this home became private, it reached similar arrangements with other nursing homes in the borough.[31] It clearly felt that the needs of the borough were being met by the voluntary sector, and that there was no need to supplement or compete with this by building a municipal home.

The municipality developed a similarly close affiliation with the local voluntary hospital, the Royal Gwent, where it used both its general and specialist facilities. The council made a regular annual contribution to the hospital – four hundred guineas in 1920 – which entitled it to appoint two representatives to the hospital's Board.[32] In addition the town's VD clinic was located at, and staffed by, the hospital. Yet this level of engagement did not result in close co-operation, or even in a particularly easy relationship between the sectors, as we show below.

Despite the fact that the council had contributed towards the cost of an extension for the treatment of VD this did not give it any direct control of the service. This was problematic not only in itself, but also because while most cases could be dealt with at the voluntary hospital, poor law cases of VD could only be treated at the Poor Law infirmary, Wooloston House (later the PAI). To complicate matters further, the scheme was governed by a contentious tripartite agreement between the hospital, Newport and

30 'Child Welfare: Newport Maternity Home', *South Wales Argus*, 11 March 1919.

31 GCRO A110. M26, M35 and M37, Maternity and Child Welfare Committee Minutes, Newport County Borough Council General Council minutes, 31 March 1919, 30 June 1928 and 31 March 1930.

32 GCRO A110. M.27, Newport Finance Committee Minutes, Newport County Borough Council General Council minutes, 28 May and 1 October 1920.

Monmouthshire County Council.[33] While it is clear that the two local authorities had difficulties co-operating, even after Monmouthshire left the agreement relations do not seem to have eased between Newport and the Royal Gwent. Despite a comment in 1926 from the municipal VD committee indicating that 'all differences' between them and the voluntary hospital had 'been settled', it took another three years for a formal agreement to be signed.[34] Even then, it appears that the matter was not completely resolved as in 1930 the committee reported it was 'still endeavouring to make satisfactory arrangements with the Royal Gwent Hospital'.[35] As the matter continued to drag on, the committee became increasingly testy in its approach to the problem:

> [We have] not been successful in persuading the authorities of the Royal Gwent Hospital to agree to the Committee's proposals for the carrying out of certain pathological work relating to Newport patients who attend the treatment centre, this in spite of the fact that the proposals are desirable and just, had been agreed by the Welsh Board of Health ... and were placed before the Hospital House Committee by a deputation.[36]

33 As early as 1924 Monmouthshire signalled its desire to withdraw from this agreement, and in the process of renegotiation it became clear that officials were unable to 'draw up a joint scheme to the satisfaction of all parties'. The unspecified 'contentious matters' were referred to the Welsh Board of Health for arbitration, and although the Board suggested a solution 'with the hope of completing the agreement,' the councils rapidly moved to a position whereby each would 'deal directly with the hospital' rather than attempting a coordinated approach. See GCRO A110. M.31 and M32, Newport Venereal Diseases Committee, Quarterly Report to the Council, Newport County Borough Council General Council minutes, 1 March 1924 and 25 May 1925.

34 GCRO, A110. M33 and M36, Newport Venereal Diseases Committee, Quarterly Report to the Council, Newport County Borough Council General Council minutes, 31 March and 28 October 1926, and 6 February and 27 April 1929.

35 GCRO, A110. M37, Maternity and Child Welfare Committee Minutes, Newport County Borough Council General Council minutes, 1 May 1930.

36 Ibid. 2 December 1930.

By 1930 then, the VD service of the town was hampered both by a failure to create a satisfactory working agreement with the voluntary hospital, and the fact that treatment in the borough was split between the Royal Gwent and the Poor Law hospital. In addition to this, the borough's MOH did not have any ability to direct the work of the Medical Officer at the voluntary hospital. In an attempt to remedy this situation and improve coordination, the MOH considered centralising the town's entire VD provision at Wooloston, and arranging for inpatient beds there in place of those at the council's disposal at the Royal Gwent.[37] However, as the PAI was never appropriated to the Public Health Committee and the clinic remained located at the Royal Gwent the level of coordination of the borough's VD provision did not improve throughout the rest of the period, with Wooloston continuing to treat only PAI patients and Gwent taking the rest. This led to continued unease in the relationship between the municipal and voluntary sectors, and the resulting service.

This lack of co-ordination was felt in the hospital services of the town more widely. The Ministry of Health inspector visiting the town in 1932 noted that there was almost no consultation going on between the Public Assistance Committee and the Gwent Hospital, despite the latter expressing willingness to co-operate.[38] The inspector also recommended that the PAI, Wooloston, be appropriated and developed, but as we have seen, this was not ultimately acted upon by the council.[39] In 1932 they were apparently considering the matter, however, since the PAI included a separate Infirmary and Hospital, which were already doing a fair range of work. However, a

37 TNA MH96/387, Survey Report, Newport, 26–8.

38 Ibid. 40–1. Representatives from the Royal Gwent had written to the council in 1929 suggesting (in the words of the Ministry inspector) 'that there might be advantage in their being represented on the PAC with a view to some coordination between their own hospital and the Poor Law institution. I was informed that this request was entirely ignored and no consultations whatever on the subject of cooperation or coordination have since taken place. This is regrettable' (41).

39 The inspector suggested that in particular, an appropriated PAI could house a more developed maternity service and artificial light treatment. Schemes for TB and VD treatment could also be brought more directly under municipal and Welsh National Memorial Association control respectively (Ibid. 38–9).

comment from the Ministry's inspector is revealing of the attitudes and inclinations of council members: 'there appear to be no insuperable difficulties [to appropriation] … though there may be local opposition on the part of certain officials of the Institution and possibly the PAC itself'.[40]

This reinforces the lack of drive to improve and expand the municipal hospital provision in the town despite the apparent willingness of the voluntary institution to act in tandem with the council. This may have been exacerbated by a fairly passive MOH, who had been acting in this role for many years by 1929 'and is inclined to wait till consulted instead of himself initiating proposals', although he had reported in favour of appropriation in principle.[41] This also removed another potential ally to any Labour drive to improve health services.

It was not simply in the areas of MCW, VD and hospital provision that the council relied heavily on voluntary services to supplement, or even largely replace, its own work. The TB service, as in the rest of Wales, was contracted out to the Welsh National Memorial Association.[42] This meant that, unlike in England where local authorities were directly responsible for dispensaries run by TB officers as well as in many cases sanatorium or hospital treatment, in Wales the Association provided the full spectrum of services apart from aftercare. It had its own sanatoria, TB officers, hospitals, and research facilities, all integrated components of the principality-wide

40 Ibid. 38.

41 Ibid. 40. The MOH, Dr Howard-Jones was due to retire in 1932, and the Ministry inspector suggested that this would be a good time to move matters forward.

42 The Welsh National Memorial Association was set up in 1910 as a voluntary organisation to combat the spread of TB in Wales. Under the 1921 Public Health (Tuberculosis) Act, local authorities were permitted to discharge their duties under it by coming to a financial arrangement with the Association. TNA MH96/1099, Newport County Borough Council: Treatment of Tuberculosis Scheme 1920–30, Circular 190 (Wales), Ministry of Health & Welsh Board of Health, 25th May 1921, confirmed that all Welsh County Boroughs and County Councils had entered into an agreement with the Association for provision of all persons suffering from TB. For a more general exploration of the Association's role in TB provision in Wales, see L. Bryder, 'The King Edward VII Welsh National Memorial Association and its Policy Towards Tuberculosis, 1910–48', *Welsh History Review*, 13:2 (1986).

organisation. While it was technically a voluntary body, the local authorities were the major contributors to its funds and had majority representation on several of its key committees. At the end of the interwar period the Report of the Enquiry into TB in Wales praised the Association for the quality of its sanatoria while also remarking upon its failure to provide a full TB service and to fully co-ordinate with local authorities.[43] And as the following discussion shows, the combined issues of lack of proper control over TB provision and its increasing cost were to prove to be ongoing sores in Newport throughout the interwar period.

In 1922 both Cardiff and Newport Borough Councils voted that the work of the TB officer and his staff, rather than being part of the Association, should come under the direct control of the respective councils' Health Committees through the local Medical Officers of Health.[44] Invited by Newport's Coordination Committee to give details of the lack of cooperation in the health services, the MOH, Dr Howard-Jones, prepared a detailed document enumerating the shortcomings of the TB service in the town. He complained that the medical work in this area was divided between three different organisations – his own department, the School Medical Service and the Welsh National Memorial Association. The practical outcome of this arrangement was that there was 'much overlapping of efforts in many directions, a large amount of unnecessary clerical work ... ignorance on the part of one dep[artmen]t in reference to the work of others, and much unnecessary work in the visitation of homes by different officials'.[45]

Howard-Jones believed that in order to create an effective department, he needed all health services centralised under his control. He argued strongly that Newport's decision to hand over control to the Association was 'contrary to the principle upon which local government is based in

43 Clement Davies, Chair of the Enquiry, quoted in Bryder, 'The King Edward VII Welsh National Memorial Association', 210–11.

44 TNA MH96/1099, Newport County Borough Council: Treatment of Tuberculosis Scheme 1920–1930, 'Letter from Newport to Board of Health, 19 June 1922'.

45 Ibid. 'Coordination of Public Health Services at Newport – Report by the MOH, Dr J. Howard Jones'.

this country', that it had reduced sensitivity to local TB problems, had unnecessarily constrained medical staff, and, overall, had led to inefficient provision. Thus while the Welsh National Memorial Association was efficient in providing institutional treatment, he argued that 'better progress would take place if local authorities carried out the detailed work themselves apart from the provision of sanatoria and Training Colonies'.[46] We have seen in the context of appropriation that the MOH was not as dynamic in practice as he was in his recommendations. However, in order to get round these problems, and to prevent the town from breaking away from the Association, in 1923 arrangements were made for the TB nurse to be moved from the Welsh National Memorial Association to the town's health department. While this was done 'in order to improve the coordination of the work,' the TB officer, however, remained under the jurisdiction of the Association.[47]

In addition to the difficulties of coordinating provision – something which was also, as we have seen, a feature of the council's relationship with the local voluntary hospital – an ongoing theme in the relationship between the town and the Association, was the feeling on the part of the council that they were not receiving good value for money. This only became more rancorous as time went on. As spending on TB began to take up an increasing proportion of the entire health budget for the town, councillors began to question the financial basis of their contributions to the Association. As early as 1925, after agreeing to fund a shortfall in the Association's income, the council made it clear that it would not be prepared to fund any future increase 'unless the basis of contribution by all local authorities is altered in such a manner as will ensure that each local authority will pay its proper proportion towards the expenses of the Association.'[48] This articulated a more general feeling that Newport was somehow paying more than its fair

46 Ibid. 'Coordination of Public Health Services at Newport – Report by the MOH, Dr J. Howard Jones'.

47 MOH Annual Report, Newport, 1923, p. 36. The plea for better aftercare facilities was also made in the Report for 1926 (p. 36) and throughout the 1930s, notably that for 1937 (p. 55).

48 GCRO A110. M12/1, Newport Health Committee Minutes, 17 February 1925.

share, something which had been first raised in the negotiations with the Board of Health and the Association in 1922.[49] The local press, while refusing to criticise the work of the Welsh National Memorial Association, was clear that it could not 'be stated that the basis of contributions as between local authorities was satisfactory.'[50]

Over the next few years the Association continued, despite such protests, to ask for more money, and following the 1929 Local Government Act a principality-wide agreement was reached, which set the level of contributions for all Welsh local authorities. Newport's annual contribution on this basis was £3952 per annum, and although Councillor Frank Quick (Labour group leader and Newport's negotiator on this matter) admitted that while this was more than the town had paid up to this point, he attempted to lessen the blow by stressing that it was 'proportionally less than the other local authorities'.[51] The result of this agreement was that while Newport council spent considerably less than the County Borough average on its TB service up to 1929, after this point its spending increased two-and-a-half fold, and throughout the 1930s the cost of its TB provision remained above the County Borough average. This change corresponds with the jump in expenditure on health in the borough illustrated in Figure 6.1. Figure 6.3 shows that the other County Boroughs in Wales followed exactly the same pattern (in contrast with the national picture for England and Wales), indicating the level to which Newport's spending was dictated by the 1929 agreement rather than by local decision making.

49 See TNA MH96/1099, Newport County Borough Council: Treatment of Tuberculosis Scheme 1920–1930, A Summary of the Proceedings of a Conference Between the Representatives of the Cardiff City Council, the Newport Town Council and Officers of the Welsh Board of Health, 4 September 1922 and Ibid. Summary of Round Table Conference on Proposed Administrative Changes to the Outpatient Work of TB in the Cardiff and Newport Areas, 11 October 1922.

50 'Newport's finances,' *South Wales Weekly Argus*, 4 September 1926.

51 The need for increases was explained as being partly the result of the Association's 'heavy financial liabilities' in providing an additional hospital in South Wales. Contributions were based 'half on population and half on the reduced (de-rated) rateable value', see A110. M12/2, Newport Health Committee Minutes, 20 August 1929.

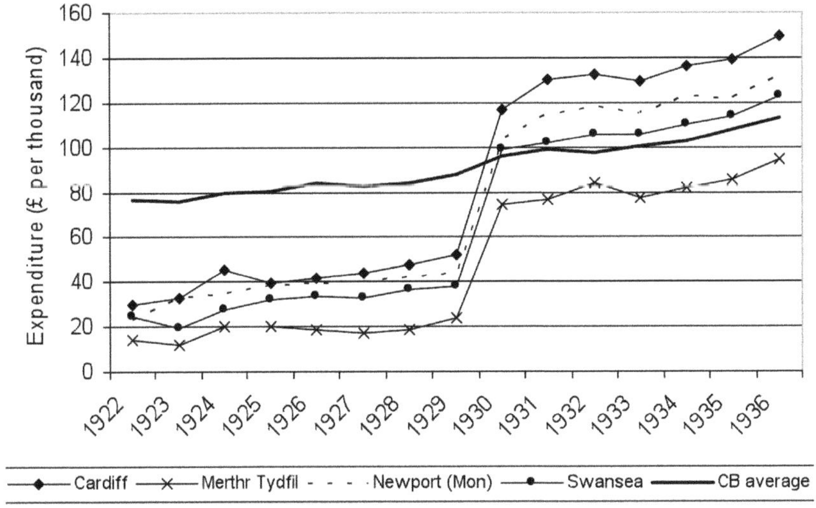

Figure 6.3 Expenditure per Thousand on TB Services in Welsh County Boroughs, 1922/3–36/7
Source: Local Government Financial statistics, 1922/3–36/7

By the end of the 1930s the amount Newport was spending on its TB scheme was a cause of considerable complaint by councillors. In 1938 the deputy chair of the Health Committee, Councillor Humphries, made a statement on the proposals of the Welsh National Memorial Association's ideas for expansion. He began by noting that over the previous eight years there had been a general increase in the spending on public health services in the town, excluding TB, of 9.6 per cent, but an increase in spending on TB of 57.7 per cent:

> we have not an unlimited amount of money to play with, and ... there must be some proportion between the expenditure ... on tuberculosis and that of other health services ... What I have said must not in any way be taken to indicate lack of sympathy with efforts to stamp out this fell disease, and certainly not as any indication that Newport wish to break away from the Memorial Association.[52]

52 'Newport View on Grants,' *South Wales Weekly Argus*, 12 February 1938.

He and other [unnamed] Newport representatives at a recent conference on the subject objected to being asked to pay a greater contribution to the Association when other local authorities had done far less to reduce poor housing or to tackle other means of decreasing the incidence of TB. They believed that they should only have to pay for 'the prevention and care of tuberculosis in their areas ... [As] local authorities can do the [preventive and aftercare] work better than the Association, and further, it is the *duty* of the respective local authorities to do such work' [emphasis in original]. Thus the entire town TB services should be handed over to municipal councils.[53] The Chair of the Finance Committee, A. E. Pugh, observing that the Health Committee would require £94,228 in the coming year, noted that the rise of £6481 was largely due to the increased demand from the Welsh National Memorial Association. He stated that 'he did not want to be niggardly about social services; but he did not want the ratepayers fleeced to satisfy any particular whim of a minority to pander to sentiment outside the council chamber, when that sentiment meant spending thousands of pounds without proof of practical value in return.'[54] Unlike West Hartlepool, which was ambivalent about spending money on services at all, here the concern seems more to have been a desire for an effective service which was fairly funded: the Welsh reliance on a voluntary association did not seem, in Newport's opinion, to offer such an opportunity.

Although the 1939 Anti-Tuberculosis in Wales report confirmed that Newport was not the only local authority to be experiencing difficulties in their relationship with the Association and with tackling TB in their area, it did little to offer any resolution.[55] There was an attempt to improve their councils' working relationship with the Association by seeking more representation on the National Board, and forming a TB Sub-Committee, consisting of all the Health Committee members – to which the Association's TB Officer was invited. The council also supported the recommen-

53 Ibid.

54 'Newport's Capital Expenditure,' *South Wales Weekly Argus*, 12 March 1938.

55 Report of the Committee of Inquiry into the Anti-Tuberculosis Service in Wales and Monmouthshire (London, 1939).

dation of the Report that a local authority could make grants in suitable cases where a TB patient voluntarily entered residential institutions.[56] However, none of these measures addressed the problem of the distorted level of investment in TB care, nor the failure of the Association's methods to tackle the deep-rooted socio-economic problems that were at the base of Wales's high TB rates. By being tied to a national-level scheme councils lost any ability to either direct the type of services provided for TB, or the amount of money such a scheme cost their ratepayers. In this sense the Welsh experience was very different from that of England, where there was no formalised nationwide voluntary organisation attempting to provide a comprehensive TB service.

So far in this section we have shown what an essential part non-municipal organisations were to the overall network of health care of Newport, with significant areas of the council's statutory health services provided via the voluntary sector. Thus, even if Newport Labour Party (or indeed any other party) had been more inclined to push the health agenda it might have been hampered by the extent to which voluntarism had colonised what was often seen as traditional Labour, or at least municipal, ground. This section also reveals however, that we should also be wary of making an automatic equation between reliance on voluntary services and reduced costs to the council. In some cases, such as in the area of MCW where voluntary contributions commonly made up over fifty per cent of the spending in milk, the money-saving implications were clear. However, in others the opposite was the case. Being part of a long term, principality-wide agreement with the Welsh National Memorial Association not only took decision making out of the hands of councillors – in stark contrast to the presumption behind interwar municipal health provision generally – but as a consequence also tied the town to disproportionate levels of expenditure. And in addition, reinforcing our findings for West Hartlepool, the problematic relationships which so often emerged as a consequence of creating and sustaining joint or outsourced services could have a lasting and negative impact on the nature and efficiency of health care provision in the town.

56 GCRO A110. M12/5, Newport Health Committee Minutes, 29 March 1939.

Consequently, we can see how relying heavily on voluntary services may have been one means by which councils could negotiate their health care responsibilities, but this path was by no means without its costs, both financial and organisational. And as we now go on to show, it could also have profound implications in terms of issues of governance. While in general we have focussed in this study on the main services provided by municipal health departments – TB, MCW, VD, infectious disease and other hospital provision – in truth the responsibilities of these departments had a much wider span. In the last part of this section we take up another example, the welfare of the blind.[57] Just as it used voluntary organisations in order to meet some of its other health service obligations, Newport council relied heavily on its local voluntary blind aid society for the delivery of these services.[58]

This area of provision is particularly pertinent for our discussion of the balance between municipal and voluntary services as it was singled out by the Ministry of Health precisely in this context. In 1934 it raised concerns over the dependence of some local authorities on voluntary associations for the discharge of their duties in relation to the blind: given the fact that they were being paid public money it felt it was not appropriate to have so little supervision.[59] Although the Ministry's reservations were not party political, some councils – and particularly Labour ones (Barnsley being a typical example) – were already in the process of taking over the functions of the voluntary societies, seeing that they were providing services more suitably discharged by a municipal authority. Indeed, we might go further to suggest that what could be thought of as an 'over reliance' on voluntary services was in direct conflict with the ideal of an active, responsible council. The Ministry's own attitude was informed by incidents such as the scandal to hit Newport's blind services in the early 1930s.

57 This was following the 1920 Blind Persons Act.

58 Blind societies tended to provide a range of services: visits by home teachers, training in a range of skills deemed suitable for the blind (typically piano tuning, weaving, basket and brush making); and often workshops where blind workers could come and make items, which were sometimes sold through a designated shop. By the late 1920s these local societies were often also the vehicle through which the council gave weekly allowances to the unemployable blind.

59 Fifteenth Annual Report of the Ministry of Health, 1933–4, Cmd. 4664, xii, p. 87.

In the 1920s, while the mechanics of the administration of the municipal blind scheme in Newport were not well thought out, the voluntary society was active and, as we might expect from this borough, well supported by the council.[60] However, by the early 1930s there were strong signs that the voluntary society was failing to provide an efficient and effective service for the blind of the borough. Admittedly, the society had a strong local profile, good at providing 'general social services' as well as being 'outstandingly successful' in raising voluntary money.[61] But in other areas a visit by a ministry inspector revealed a number of serious shortcomings, with her report implying that the council used voluntary organisations more out of convenience than as a matter of principle.[62] Matters came to a head in the autumn of 1933 when a number of irregularities came to light, notably the embezzlement of an unknown sum of money (estimated at £1000), poor and inaccurate book keeping, and an over-dominance of the secretary, who might be kindly described as eccentric.[63] The report emphasised the failure of supervision on the part of either of the local authorities which

60 The Board of Health inspector found that the Health Committee was responsible for the blind scheme, but for the purposes of the Act it had no co-opted members, nor were any Guardians on the Committee. Newport countered this criticism by replying that a member of the Health Committee was also a Guardian, and that two other members of the Health Committee were on the Management Committee of the Newport and Monmouthshire Blind Aid Society. It therefore felt that it was unnecessary to co-opt any members. See TNA MH96/61, Newport Blind Services Correspondence, 1925–33, Newport County Borough Council: Scheme in Relation to the Blind Persons Act 1920, minutes by Mr Thurman, Board of Health, 12 September 1925 and Newport Town Clerk to Ministry of Health, 22 October 1925.

61 TNA MH96/61, Newport Blind Services Correspondence, 1925–33, Newport County Borough Council: Scheme in Relation to the Blind Persons Act 1920, Report on the Blind Welfare Services of Newport County Borough, Winifred Bramhall, 14 September 1931.

62 Ibid. 12.

63 TNA MH96/62, Blind Services in Newport, 1934–8, notes of meeting between Ministry of Health officials and N. T. J. Moses, Borough Treasurer of Newport, 22 March 1934; and TNA MH96/61, Newport Blind Services Correspondence, 1925–33, Newport County Borough Council: Scheme in Relation to the Blind Persons Act 1920, letter from J. K. Price, emergency acting chair of the Blind Aid Society, to Miss Bramhall, 25 November 1933. Price's letter, which set out in bald terms the short-

used the society. It found that the two Monmouthshire County Council representatives did not attend any of the Blind Aid Society's Committee meetings in 1933–4, while the four Newport representatives put in a total of six attendances between them.[64] Unsurprisingly, the report found that the Committee was: 'incompetent in administering the important duties and responsibilities devolving upon the Society ... They failed to exercise proper control over the staff, and the fundamental principles of financial control were ignored'.[65]

The ongoing failings revealed by the inspector demonstrate the dangers of using a voluntary organisation to discharge the functions of the council. While making no claims for the efficiency of council services, nor suggesting that the administration of the health department was infallible, council affairs were much more closely scrutinised and subject to checks. For an individual's judgement to hold sway (as the MOH Dr Willoughby's did in Eastbourne), the majority of the council had to be happy to allow it, while financial mismanagement as we saw in Barnsley was eventually discovered because of the system of auditing, Voluntary organisations, and particularly small ones, could be amateurish, dominated by one or two individuals and as the above example demonstrated, were better able to evade checks and balances if they so desired. The combination of a negligent supervisory committee, an unpopular secretary and a dishonest chief clerk ensured that the blind services of both Newport and Monmouthshire were moribund for much of the 1930s. Voluntary organisations may have been able to deliver services on behalf of the council; they may even have been supported by local users; but they did not necessarily do it either more cheaply or better than the health department.

comings of the Society was written from his home address, headed by the comment, 'don't think I would send a letter from the office like this'.

64 TNA MH96/62, Blind Services in Newport, 1934–8, Newport County Borough Council: Scheme in Relation to the Blind Persons Act 1920, Report of Sub-Committee Appointed by Joint Meeting of Representatives of Newport Corporation and Monmouthshire County Council to Enquire in to the Administration of the Newport and Monmouthshire Blind Aid Society, September 1934 (Strictly Private and Confidential – not for publication.), 2.

65 Ibid.

Conclusions

As with our other case study boroughs a detailed examination of the archives in Newport reveals a level of complexity not suggested in the national-level data analysed in Chapters Two and Three of this book. Higher than average levels of Labour representation on the council did not translate into actual power, for example: one year's control of the Health Committee resulted in the founding of a smallpox hospital, suggesting that the Labour Party acted when it could, but the strong ethos of voluntarism hampered much of its expansion in the field of health service development. Similarly, above-average levels of expenditure for part of the period have been revealed to have based on enforced investment in one service – TB – which was administered outside the borough.

However, while the case study has added greatly to our understanding of the borough's development of health services, questions remain unanswered. For example, the archives do not provide firm evidence for the reasons behind Labour's lack of demonstrable interest in promoting the health services of the borough. We might reasonably tie this to an established ethos of (upper) middle class voluntarism which had colonised and de-politicised health (and particularly MCW) services; voluntarism having had a longer history than municipalism. It is interesting to contrast Newport's position with that of Barnsley where the voluntary hospital, through its association with the miners, became tied to specifically Labour concerns rather than being in opposition to them. Such a comparison allows us to show that not only could local Labour parties have very different characteristics which had a significant impact on their priorities, but equally voluntary provision could be diverse and carry with it vastly different social meanings. We do not know whether the Labour Party in Newport also saw itself as allied with the various voluntary efforts – this would not be inconsistent with Labour ideology or indeed practice in other locales. However, if they were, they were silent on the matter. Nonetheless, however one-sided the status quo in the field of health care was, it seems that it was adequate: although the Ministry of Health inspector in 1932 recommended greater co-ordination between voluntary and municipal sectors, and the appropriation of the Infirmary part of the PAI, relations with Whitehall were generally unstrained.

Overall, examining the council's association with voluntary bodies revealed the tortuous and problematic nature of many of these relationships, which almost without fail saw institutional interests put before efficiency, retarding the quality and speed of service provision. More than this, the example of the blind society reveals the depth of problems which could develop in the absence of proper regulation and supervision. Similarly, the borough's relationship with the Welsh National Memorial Association sets the issue of voluntarism in a much wider framework and ties it very obviously to a national framework. While its difficulties with the Association in the 1930s were clearly centred on the expensive nature of its provision, in the early 1920s it seems particularly evident that the borough was trying to take control of its own affairs and to ensure a united and efficient TB service. Not only does the impact of the Association on the council's spending emphasise the importance of taking into account the distinctively 'Welsh' experience of Newport in this matter, but it also raises a broader point. At a time of arch municipalism, the difficulties and expense involved in scaling up provision beyond a local level illustrate forcefully the extent to which some County Boroughs wanted to have absolute control over the direction of their resources and their services. This in turn reminds us of the *volte face* represented by the passing of the National Health Service Act, and the very different context from which it emerged.

CHAPTER SEVEN

West Hartlepool

West Hartlepool, in contrast with our other case studies, had none of the characteristics which would predict high levels of spending on health. It was quite poorly off, Labour had little sway on its council, and it was in a depressed area of the country which meant that it had many other pressing social problems as well as healthcare. True to this predicted form, it did not invest particularly highly in its municipal health services. This chapter will set out the range of factors which underpinned this low level of investment, highlighting again how far predictions at the aggregate level must be joined with local observations. In particular, in West Hartlepool, they must be considered alongside the generally parsimonious outlook of the council over a fairly long period of time – but one that achieved positive outcomes as well as poor ones.

West Hartlepool lies four miles north of the Tees estuary in County Durham, north-east England. Finally joined with neighbouring Hartlepool in 1967, the town originally sprang up in the 1840s following the granting of a charter to West Hartlepool Dock Company to build rival docks to the south west of the old town of Hartlepool. West Hartlepool borough grew rapidly around the new docks and quickly overshadowed the old town, and by 1900 the combined Hartlepools port had become one of the four busiest in the country. Shipbuilding was hard hit by the 1930s depression, however, as were interconnected industries such as marine engine manufacture, and this decade saw the permanent closure of some of the dockyards. At the depth of the depression in 1931, shipbuilding was described as having 'almost come to a standstill,' with engine building 'scarcely any better,' and the docks were also handling fewer imports and exports. This led the Ministry of Health inspector when he visited the town in 1931 to observe that the town was 'one of the "black" areas as regards unemployment', which was 'nearly double that of County Boroughs as a whole'.[1]

The town similarly recorded above-average infant mortality levels up to 1936, as well as experiencing high rates of deaths from TB. The 1931 Ministry of Health survey noted in relation to the latter that there was 'still considerable overcrowding in the borough, and this factor, with the prolonged industrial depression, may possibly be responsible for the higher death rate'. This same report found low levels of spending in virtually every area of the municipal health service (illustrated in Figure 7.1): the health visitor staff was described as 'barely adequate', TB provision was 'not satisfactory'. And yet, as we discuss in this chapter, West Hartlepool was not necessarily as poor as it made out, with its parsimony the result of more than lack of funds: certainly the Ministry of Health felt that for a long time 'economy was practised too much at the expense of the public health services'.[2]

We have already noted that the town was relatively poorly off: its rateable property values were consistently below the national average and only very slightly above Barnsley's. The rate of tax it actually set in the pound averaged out at the same as the national level over the whole period, but it showed a very different pattern over time: higher in the early years, but then failing to keep pace after 1929, and even undergoing a series of cuts subsequently.[3] This contrasts particularly sharply with Barnsley, where rates were raised significantly from the mid-1920s. Setting a low rate in the pound does not necessarily indicate a lack of investment, of course. It could reflect an improvement in social conditions which meant that council services were less relied upon. Given West Hartlepool's socio-economic indicators in the midst of the depression, however, this seems to be too generous an interpretation. Instead the falling rate in the pound probably reflected a growing opposition to further spending, and a desire to keep ratepayers happy by maintaining low taxes.

1 TNA MH66/988, Survey Report, West Hartlepool.

2 TNA MH66/988, Survey Report, West Hartlepool, 1,3–4 and 68. In 1931 (the year of the Ministry survey) the infant mortality rate had been above average for seven years out of the previous nine, and in 1922, 1925, 1927 and 1929 it had been especially high (100 per thousand or more), mainly due to the prevalence of respiratory diseases and influenza.

3 See Chapter 3, Figure 3.7b and e.

The reluctance of the council to spend was not reserved simply for its health services but was spread across the board. As R. Wilson has argued, in West Hartlepool the 'political response was not to need, rather it was to what the policy of "economy and efficiency" would allow.'[4] For example, Ministry officials visiting the borough in the early 1930s found an 'exceptional degree' of overcrowding, and yet the council made little use of the Housing Acts to engage in slum clearance or construction of municipal estates until the late 1930s, leaving private enterprise to provide the bulk of new housing.[5]

The political colour of the borough can be summed up in the words of the first Labour councillor to be elected, on the occasion of his maiden speech in 1919: 'I can understand to a limited extent the feelings of Daniel when he was thrust into the lions' den.'[6] Indeed, as we will show throughout this chapter, West Hartlepool's municipal politics were dominated to varying degrees across the whole period by 'business-minded' independents who understood their main duty to be to keep rates down, rather than to expand the range of services provided by the council. For much of the 1920s this single Labour councillor's position was not much improved, as the party held only a handful of seats. Newspaper reports suggest that this was due in part to internal divisions within the party, but was also – in stark contrast to Barnsley – the product of divisions between the local trade unions and the town's Labour Party.[7] Councillor (later Alderman) Turnbull, who was a central figure in the local Engineers' Union for forty years, strongly opposed any links between trade unionism and socialism, and worked on the principle that politics should play no part in council decision making.[8] However, from November 1936 Labour was able to construct a working majority on the council, and although we lack the

4 R. Wilson, 'The Economy, Housing and Health in West Hartlepool, 1919–1939', MPhil thesis, University of Teesside, no date.

5 TNA MH66/988, Survey Report, West Hartlepool, Memo produced by the Ministry relating to the Poole Joint Sanatorium Committee (n.d).

6 'Vacant Sites,' *Northern Daily Mail*, 5 November 1919.

7 See 'An Abominable Mess,' *Northern Daily Mail*, 30 October 1933; 'Mrs Thompson's Position,' *Northern Daily Mail*, 31 October 1933.

8 'Stormy Scenes at West Hartlepool Town Council Meeting,' *Northern Daily Mail*, 8 November 1933.

financial statistics to quantify any change in spending that resulted from this political shift, as we show below, it was accompanied by an upsurge in activity within the council's health services.

In this chapter we will explore not only what the council's general stinting approach meant in terms of day-to-day delivery of services, but also how this interacted with other factors in the borough to produce the picture we see in the expenditure data. What the local records reveal is an interaction between the undoubted parsimony of a strong body of the town's councillors and the competing interests of other health service providers: GPs, voluntary hospitals and other local authorities. And in addition, in common with our other case study areas, we also show the importance of a range of micro-factors – such as the personality of individual doctors and clinic staff – in determining the use and success of municipal facilities. Consequently, what we see is that the explanation for the slow development of services and infrastructure in the borough cannot be simply attributed to a 'stinting' council, which we discuss in the first part of the chapter. Equally significantly, in the second half of the chapter we show how the dynamic interaction of the priorities of different interest groups – including a parsimonious council – could produce positive outcomes as well as retard progress.

Problematising the 'Poor Stinting Council'

The first thing we should note in our caution against writing off West Hartlepool as straightforwardly poor and stinting is the non-static nature of its economic profile. We noted at the start of this chapter that it was hard hit by economic decline, and had low rateable values throughout the period. However, by 1935 the visiting Ministry of Health inspector recorded a 'slight improvement'. This had been enabled by the town winning some international shipping contracts, an increase in iron and steel work, and 'partly the result of increase in dock work with [the] lift in the timber trade'.[9] Equally,

9 TNA MH66/993, Resurvey Report, West Hartlepool, 1.

the docks, which were the third largest local employer and dealt with coal and timber exports, were by then recovering relatively quickly from their depression. This revival in the town's employment prospects was aided by the fact that the 1920s had seen the town's economy becoming increasingly diversified.[10] As a result, West Hartlepool had a different experience of the depression than the rest of Co. Durham, where the depression lasted much longer, and where the economy was generally less diversified. By 1937 the town had one of the best recovery rates in the country.[11]

This suggests that we might need to complicate our understanding of the borough as 'poor'. The relative difference of its economy to that of the surrounding region was noted by Whitehall in the late 1930s when, it was awarded a lower level of grant than other towns designated as having 'Special Area' status.[12] More than this, the Ministry of Health felt that the unemployment figures produced for the area were actually 'misleading' because the Ministry of Labour returns were for both the Hartlepools. Ministry of Health officials felt that the Borough of Hartlepool was 'down and out but West Hartlepool County Borough's much better off. The rates are lower than last year, but apart from this we do not know how far things have altered'. As a result they stated that 'so far as we know there are no special difficulties in the Town Council's financial position'.[13] This is not

10 This range of industries included a paper and saw mill, timber and creosoting plants, the manufacture of mesh for reinforced concrete and the largest de-tinning works in the country. A Cerebos plant was also opened which produced salt, Bisto, jellies, blancmanges and custard powder. This expansion had also increased the managerial and professional classes of the town. Wilson, 'Economy, Housing and Health', 54.

11 Ibid., 66.

12 In relation to grants for the building of the Poole Joint Sanatorium (see below), the Special Areas Expenditure Committee felt that it was unfair that West Hartlepool and South Shields both got 50 per cent contributory grants owing to the 'considerable difference in the financial situations of the two County Boroughs. See TNA MH61/30, Commissioners for the Special Areas, 1935–48, minute, 27 September 1937.

13 TNA, MH66/991, Survey Correspondence, West Hartlepool, Ministry of Health, Minute Ward to Wrigley, 15 February 1932, and further note 24 February 1932. For example, in 1934 while the percentage of insured jobless in West Hartlepool was 29.8 per cent, in Hartlepool it stood at 44.5 per cent. See D. E. Wallace, *Reports of Investigations into the Industrial Conditions in Certain Depressed Areas, Part II, Durham and Teesside* (London, 1934) Table 1, p. 116.

to make any claim for the prosperity of the town, and certainly in relation to the country as a whole it was poor and hit hard by the economic recession. However, it is important to note that relative to the other towns of the north-east, it was able to rise more rapidly out of the slump.

This forms part of the backdrop to the development of the town's health services: in both the early 1920s and after 1935 the town had a greater potential to pay for the development of its health services. Our ability to fully analyse spending for these periods is limited by the fact that the Registrar-General's statistics only cover the years 1922/3–36/7 – and it was the years outside those dates when most of the health service expansion seems to have occurred in West Hartlepool. Therefore any sense of the development of the council's services in these years has to be gleaned from a range of sources including the council minutes and reports from the local paper, the *Northern Daily Mail*.

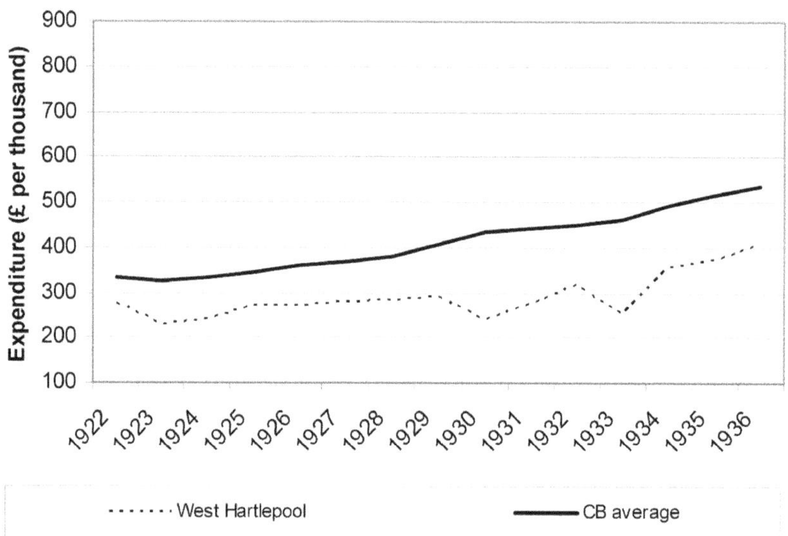

Figure 7.1 Expenditure per Thousand on Health, West Hartlepool County Borough, 1922/3–36/7
Source: Local Government Financial statistics, 1922/23–36/7

For the period for which we have figures, however, it is quite clear that West Hartlepool spent significantly under the County Borough average on its health services (Figure 7.1). On one level this is explained by the dominance of a self-consciously economising group of councillors, who have been described by Wilson as forming a 'business party' on the council for the majority of the 1920s and the first half of the 1930s. The 1920s saw the gradual creeping dominance of anti-spenders, meaning that there is no single date to which we can point to show that a critical mass of like-minded anti-spend councillors took over the council. All we can really say is that by 1926–7 they seem to have been in the majority.[14] From then until the mid-1930s there was little or no debate on issues of health service expenditure, largely because there were so few schemes brought forward to arouse controversy. Undoubtedly West Hartlepool was adversely affected by the general strike of 1926 and the prolonged coal strike, but the economies the strikes introduced were exaggerated by the consolidation of power of anti-spend councillors who were reluctant to make even the smallest investments in their services. During this period council candidates in favour of 'municipal enterprise, public schemes for the unemployed and a Workers' Charter' were defeated in local elections, with ratepayer concerns over keeping spending low acting as the main political force.[15] The Ministry of Health in the early 1930s, found there to be a 'stupid and ... obstinate resistance of a powerful section of the Council' to health service development at this time.[16]

Relations between West Hartlepool council and the Ministry of Health were consequently characterised by tension caused by the council's unwillingness to expand its health services, and the Ministry's (and then the Special Areas Commissioner's) refusal to recognise West Hartlepool's claims of poverty. The impact of the dominance of the business party led the Ministry of Health to believe that the reluctance of the council to spend on services was the result, not of poverty, but of a particular state

14 It may be that the shift in attitude on the council reflected a move away from the dominance of a local Liberal elite to a 'shopocracy' more concerned with rates than wider social obligations. However, it has not yet been possible to undertake this research on the social background of councillors.

15 Wilson, 'The Economy, Housing and Health', 74–5.

16 TNA MH66/993, Resurvey Report, West Hartlepool, 5. The 'stupid and' is crossed out in the report, but is still clearly legible.

of mind. In 1932 officials observed that although there was substantial unemployment locally, the town had done quite well out of the block grant introduced under the 1929 Local Government Act. Regardless of this, expenditure on health was:

> abnormally low compared with that on other services, though these are all well below average, and the standard attained does not suggest that any exceptionally good value for money is being obtained for the money which is spent ... *the health services were starved in the days when the town was prosperous* [emphasis added].[17]

While this comment perhaps unfairly ignored the efforts made in the town before 1921 (which we discuss below) and the fact that the area had not experienced 'prosperity' for some years before the onset of the depression, it nevertheless reveals the council's reluctance to spend even given the context of the economic difficulties. It also illustrates a contrast with the situation in Newport, where some explanation for levels of investment in health was offered by the heavier spending on housing. Indeed, the scheduling of a resurvey of West Hartlepool's health services in 1935 was the Ministry of Health's reaction to the council's 'dilatory' response to the original report. Whitehall officials believed that this had been 'considered by the Council, who, with few regrets (if not with positive satisfaction) deferred all action on grounds of economy'.[18] The negligent attitude of councillors to their health services was repeatedly emphasised in this resurvey, which frequently made reference to how local medical officers faced an uphill struggle in their battle to improve the town's health services:

> [The Medical Officer of Health] has undoubtedly had a very difficult Council to deal with, and it was not altogether surprising to find ... that he had not made much headway in the intervening years. Although his energy has abated to some extent, he has kept to his programme of reforms, and seems to have had sufficient determination to wear down the ['stupid and' deleted] obstinate resistance of a powerful section of the Council, and has succeeded in getting some of the reforms which he set out to obtain when he was first appointed.[19]

17 TNA, MH66/991, Survey Correspondence, West Hartlepool, Ministry of Health Minute by Ward, 25 February 1932.
18 TNA MH66/993, Resurvey Report, West Hartlepool, 3.
19 Ibid. 5.

The Ministry's belief that the council was determined to reduce spending on all services, including health services, to the barest minimum was not simply the product of a liberal bureaucratic elite based in Whitehall and far removed from the daily realities of the 1930s depression: the tactics of the council were confirmed by a deputation from the town to the Commissioner for the Special Areas in 1937. The town's representatives admitted that rates were low, and that they had been artificially kept at 10s. 6d. in the pound for many years: 'They pleaded that their rates were artificially low and in order to keep them at their present level they had not only used up the whole of the increase in the block grant (£25,000) but had raided their balances'.[20]

This action had subsidised the rates by about a shilling a year. Alderman Hyde explained that the policy of the council, 'for a number of years had been to keep the rates down with the object of attracting industry, but they had not been particularly successful in that respect and now they find themselves faced with many deficiencies in their services'. As a result the Board of Education was harassing the council to approve an education building and development programme costing £200,000, the result of not having built an elementary school in the town for over thirty years. This statement makes it clear that the council had not only been starving its health services, but had adopted a similar policy across the board in order to reduce expenditure.

> The impression gained from the conversation with the deputation was that the council has starved their services even when they were in a position to carry out necessary works and now that they were confronted with the task of meeting the accumulated deficiencies arising from their own deliberate action they look to the Commissioner to help them out of their difficulties.[21]

Broadly then West Hartlepool council did maintain abnormally low levels of spending throughout the main part of our period, and this was associated with the dominance of an anti-spend group on the council that limited

20 TNA, MH61/30, Commissioners for the Special Areas, 1935–48, Minute on West Hartlepool Deputation, 3 November 1937. The deputation consisted of Alderman Hyde, the Town Clerk and the Borough Treasurer.

21 Ibid.

expenditure wherever and whenever possible. However, if we now turn to focus on two areas of municipal health provision in particular – MCW and TB – we can see the importance of tempering this understanding with close attention to periodisation. Archival evidence suggest that the years before 1924 and after 1936 saw far higher levels of activity and investment than suggested in the Financial Returns for the central part of the period.

In common with the nation as a whole, the immediate post-war years saw a major expansion in council MCW in West Hartlepool. An infant welfare centre was opened in Mill House in 1918, with another three following in 1920,[22] and two years later the council opened its maternity home, Grantully. Soon after the home was opened, it was expanded further and was provided with an isolation unit, while an antenatal clinic was established in town. Similarly the numbers of health visitors increased from two in 1918 to seven by 1920, and their work was reorganised to make them more effective.[23] In general during this period the council concurred with the sentiments of the single Labour councillor who believed that '[o]ne of the most important things the Council has to do at the present time ... is to see that nursing and expectant mothers are properly looked after ... [They] are responsible for the future generation ... It is money well spent'.[24]

A Ministry inspector visiting the town's MCW services in 1926, after several years of sustained investment, felt the council was doing 'good work' under their scheme, and particularly commended 'their efforts to provide for the care of expectant mothers by the appointment of a nurse for ante-natal work', and the opening of an antenatal clinic in town.[25] This essentially retrospective report reflected the achievements of the past few years of modest, but sustained, investment, and suggests that in the early

22 MOH Annual Report, West Hartlepool, 1920, p. 86.

23 Ibid. 75. The Health Visitors were reorganised so that rather than their work overlapping, one Health Visitor was assigned to a particular ward where she conducted all the visiting.

24 'High Apostle of Economy,' *Northern Daily Mail*, 5 October 1921.

25 TNA, MH66/990, Survey Appendices, West Hartlepool, Maternity and Child Welfare Report. Dr Turnbull of the Ministry of Health had visited and reported on these services in report dated 27 July 1926.

years of the interwar period the developments in West Hartlepool's MCW services were not significantly out of line with those in other boroughs.

The TB service in these early years saw a similar, if not greater, level of activity, with different parts of the service brought together into a coordinated scheme. As the MOH stated in his report of 1918: '[p]ractically all of the patients had more than one form of treatment. Sanatorium treatment after observation at the dispensary is usually followed by dispensary treatment'.[26] Health visitors actively sought out TB patients and as well as giving them advice such as keeping windows open, they reported on sufferers' home circumstances to the After Care Committee to procure them more help if necessary. A shelter colony was also established after the council took over eight huts from the West Hartlepool Society for the Prevention of Tuberculosis. In addition, this period saw the council approving an open air school for susceptible children, farm colony treatment for boys with mild cases of TB, an arrangement with the local voluntary hospital for use of its X-ray facilities, and a dental service for TB sufferers paid for by the council.[27] In 1920, the shelter scheme was extended, and while this does not appear to have gone well, this was not the result of a lack of local authority investment, but due to the unpopularity of the treatment.[28]

However as we have suggested, by the mid-1920s the balance within the council was shifting away from any willingness to spend on its services, and this had a significant impact on the development of both MCW and TB services. By the late 1920s the infant welfare centres, for example, which were held in rented church halls and had received no investment or improvements since their inception, were becoming increasingly inadequate: the one held in Alice Street, for example, was difficult to 'carry on in a satisfactory manner, more so during the colder months' owing to the

26 MOH Annual Report, West Hartlepool, 1918, pp. 53–4.

27 Teesside Archives CB/WH/C2/203, West Hartlepool Joint Consultative Committee on Tuberculosis Minutes, 1914–1927, 20 March, 24 April and 22 May 1919.

28 Ibid. 20 May 1920 and 20 June 1920. A month after the colony opened it was necessary to buy a new set of bed linen and towels for the shelters to 'replace those stolen'. It was also necessary to replace the caretaker at the shelters, as the original one, a patient, had died.

large numbers of cases attending and the lack of waiting room.[29] As a result the centres saw a decline in attendances, suggesting that women regarded them as not useful enough to use regularly. This attitude was also shared by the MOH, Dr Lilico, who felt that it would 'benefit both mother and child more to spend the afternoon on a fine summer's day down on the sands than awaiting their time at the centre'.[30]

In March 1927 the council decided 'in view of the general economic position of the district to introduce a comprehensive scheme for the reduction of staff and salaries including *inter alia* a reduction of the health visiting staff.' While the Ministry of Health refused to agree to this reduction, arguing that the borough in fact needed more rather than fewer health visitors, 'the question of an increase was not pursued.'[31] This meant that the health visiting service continued to be understaffed and underpaid.[32] The effect was twofold; the number of visits that health visitors paid actually decreased in the late 1920s, and there was a steady haemorrhaging of health visiting staff who left to find more lucrative work elsewhere, with replacements difficult to find. The central years of our period, 1926–31, when there were thirteen resignations in the borough (compared to two in Newport and one in Barnsley in the same period), is one indication of the impact low investment had on the health department's staff. This was something recognised by councillors in a debate on the matter in 1928, when Councillor Morgan asserted that 'West Hartlepool has been blackballed

29 MOH Annual Report, West Hartlepool, 1928, p. 17.

30 Ibid. 18.

31 TNA MH66/990, Survey Appendices, West Hartlepool, Maternity and Child Welfare Report.

32 The immediate post war years saw the council adopting the Local Government Board recommended scale for health visitor salaries, but by the mid 1920s it was attracting criticism from both the Ministry of Health and the professional organisation representing health visitors. This prompted the council to agree that final salaries could be increased to £193 after three years' service, if women were in possession of the correct qualifications. However, a Ministry minute in 1931 noted that the 'maximum salary paid to H[ealth] V[isitor]s in West Hartlepool in 1929 was £200 per annum, which in many places is the minimum'. See TNA MH66/988 Ministry of Health Survey, West Hartlepool, Ministry minute, 13 July 1931. Newport's final salary at this time was £222pa.

because you pay less here than in other parts of the country', a point which was reinforced by the unfavourable comparison between the terms offered by the town and those in adverts they appeared alongside.[33]

For the TB service these middle years were also ones of stagnation. In 1925 the shelter colony closed, partly because of under use, but it was not replaced by other residential accommodation, while the voluntary after-care committee (part-funded by the council) suspended a major part of its extra-nourishment programme owing to lack of funds.[34] The limited development of both the town service and sanatorium provision by 1931 was revealed in a minute by the Ministry inspector, Dr Chapman, who stated that the 'the council have no facilities to offer.' The MOH of the time, Dr McKeggie, reinforced the inadequacy of the existing infrastructure, describing the dispensary as 'dark and dirty and devoid of equipment, beyond a pair of scales and a stethoscope.'[35] The absence of X-ray apparatus meant that local doctors did not bother to send their patients to the dispensary (a trend which echoes the situation in Eastbourne). Dr Chapman also observed that the town had no sanatorium facilities so patients were sent to Newcastle, where the facilities tended to be overcrowded at certain times of the year. This shortage was exacerbated by lack of voluntary sanatoria across the whole of the north-east.[36]

While these examples (which could be multiplied across West Hartlepool's other municipal health services) show the limited and unattractive facilities which resulted from the council's unwillingness to invest in its health services in the central years of the interwar period, to write off the

33 This point is lent further weight by a comparison with boroughs like Eastbourne: Alderman Hyde argued that 'health resorts and other places were not burdened with rates as West Hartlepool was could offer bigger salaries, and naturally people applied for these bigger salaries.' '"Blackballed" by Nurses?', *Northern Daily Mail*, 8 March 1928.

34 Teesside Archives CB/WH/C2/203, West Hartlepool Tuberculosis Committee Minutes, 1914–1927, 22 June 1925 and MOH Annual Report, West Hartlepool, 1925, pp. 37–40.

35 TNA MH66/988, Survey Report, West Hartlepool, 7.

36 TNA MH66/990, Survey Appendices, West Hartlepool, Minute by Dr Chapman on the TB services, 4 February 1931.

council simply as a 'low-Labour stinter' ignores both the early developments, and those made in the final years of the period. In part, as with the earlier period of expansion, this investment was stimulated by an improved national economic situation that prompted the Ministry of Health to encourage spending on health services. So, for example, with the passing of the 1936 Midwives Act and an injunction the following year to local authorities to remove 'arbitrary restrictions or limitations on the supply of milk to mothers and young children who need extra nourishment', the Ministry of Health signalled that investment in the MCW services were both desirable and appropriate.[37]

However, these developments can also be tied closely to Labour's gaining of council control in West Hartlepool from late 1936; something which was made explicit in the debates of the time, and which supports our hypothesis of the importance of the political complexion of the council in explaining the provision of municipal health services. As the local paper reflected in November 1936:

> The Labour Party will now have an opportunity to carry out the promises they have made for better administration and progressive development. In their election manifesto they asserted the Moderates had adopted a 'do nothing' policy, and that they had exercised a stranglehold on many schemes of improvement. In recent years the development of the town has certainly not kept pace with the talk in the Council chamber ... The Labour Party have a number of ... ambitious schemes in hand – some of them highly desirable.[38]

37 Under the 1936 Act local authorities had a duty to provide an 'adequate number' of full time, salaried midwives to attend women at home, and also a system of maternity nursing for women at home. The aim of the Act was to ensure all women had access to a midwife, even if they were having a home birth. In Circular 1519, issued 1 April 1937, local authorities were asked to review their milk supply regulations and it was also suggested that, 'without departing from the principle of recovering from recipients such part of the cost as they could reasonably afford to pay, the Authorities should satisfy themselves that their scales of income are not such as to debar any mothers form taking advantage of the arrangements'. Eighteenth Annual Report of the Ministry of Health, 1936–7, Cmd. 5516, viii, 17–18.

38 Editorial 'Municipal Elections,' *Northern Daily Mail*, 3 November 1936. The new councillors were Aldermen Mason, Boanson, Clarkson and Watt.

This makes clear the Labour association with the development of social and welfare services, here made explicit in their own election promises. In fact Labour only gained control of the council through securing the cooperation of key independent councillors, but it seems to have managed this through its promise of change. Councillor Marcus Bloom stated that he was voting with Labour because: 'We want change in West Hartlepool. We can't do worse, we might do better. I support this because I believe it is for the good government of the town.'[39] The new attitude of the council was articulated by the leader of the Labour group, Alderman Lupton: 'We must stop this finicking about – doing a little bit today and a little bit tomorrow. We must get on with the job and make a success of it.' He was supported by his colleague Councillor Habron:

> This town has always been depressed. If a doctor went to visit his patients with a face like some people have whenever they talk about West Hartlepool, the patients would die right away. West Hartlepool has got to be taken away from depression and the state of mind that creates depression.[40]

This period of Labour control subsequently saw the creation of a full midwifery service for the town, with the council engaging twelve midwives and developing a new consultant obstetric service for the ante- and post-natal schemes. A panel of consultants was appointed, based at the teaching hospital in Newcastle, where women could go to for examinations. The Public Health Committee also designed an emergency service for women in labour.[41] Telephones were installed in each midwife's residence and connected with the exchange at the Grantully maternity home, so that anyone needing a midwife simply had to contact the home.[42] This development

39 Labour Takes its Revenge,' *Northern Daily Mail*, 4 December 1936.

40 'Council Intent on Two-Pool Bath,' *Northern Daily Mail*, 5 February 1937. This particular council meeting resulted in approving two municipal baths and described proposals to build two senior schools and a nursery school.

41 Teesside Archives CB/WH/C2/183, West Hartlepool Health Committee Minutes, 14 December 1936.

42 MOH Annual Report, West Hartlepool, 1937, pp. 12–14. A scale of fees and remissions for midwives' and maternity nurses' services was drawn up – £2 for midwife

provoked the remaining anti-spend councillors to make accusations of profligacy: Alderman Hyde complained that 'we shall be asked to supply them with motor-cars next' while Councillor Hogg stated 'I had to run for the doctor when my children were born. Why cannot these people do the same?'[43]

At the same time the town's TB service saw an upsurge in activity, as the dispensary was moved to the voluntary Cameron Hospital, where it enjoyed better surroundings and facilities, including (finally) close proximity to X-ray apparatus.[44] Institutional care for early and advanced cases was provided when a TB pavilion was opened at the town's isolation hospital in 1938 at a cost of just over £7000.[45] In September 1936 the MOH was empowered to provide extra nourishment to TB cases, and the number of patients covered under this scheme increased rapidly to the extent that the following year the Ministry of Health wrote protesting that the numbers were far in excess of the amount provided for in the council's expenditure estimates.[46] In the same letter the Ministry also noted that the council were sending more people to sanatoria than they had budgeted for. At the same time the council finally decided to become part of a joint scheme to create an orthopaedic hospital to the north of Durham city.[47]

Consequently our understanding of West Hartlepool as a 'stinter' needs to be tempered by an acceptance that the town saw considerable growth in services at the beginning and end of the period. Undoubtedly however, for the central years of the interwar period the municipal health

---

attendance, and £1 for employing a maternity nurse for the first week (with 10s. for subsequent weeks). There was, however, a considerable income-related subsidy, which also took into account the number of dependent children.

43 'Telephones for Midwives', *Northern Daily Mail*, 4 June 1937.

44 Teesside Archives CB/WH/C2/184, West Hartlepool Health Committee Minutes, 25 January 1937.

45 Ibid. 1 February 1937.

46 Ibid. 21 September 1936 and 22 November 1937. In 1937, 119 patients received £514 worth of food. Sanatorium treatment was received by ninety-five cases, increased from sixty-two the year before, at an increased cost of £1000. See MOH Annual Report, West Hartlepool, 1937, p. 30.

47 Teesside Archives CB/WH/C2/184, West Hartlepool Health Committee Minutes, 25 October 1937.

services were limited and slowly developing, underpinned by an extreme reluctance to raise rates and invest for the future. Nevertheless, despite this qualification, it is fair to characterise this central part of the interwar period as one that best fits the 'low Labour low spender' designation, one that resulted in visible under-investment in the health services, and that supports our hypothesis of the importance of the political complexion of the council in understanding health provision. In the following section we add a further layer to this understanding of council decisions by arguing that the pattern of the town's health services was also crucially dependent on relations with the other health service providers in the area.

Relations With Other Health-Care Bodies

The most significant of the other interests in the field of municipal health were the Ministry of Health itself, the two voluntary hospitals in the town – Cameron Hospital and Hartlepools Hospital – and (in certain cases) the surrounding local authorities. In this section we use the cases of the isolation hospital provision and attempts to work with the voluntary hospitals over the appropriation of the PAI to reveal the importance of such relationships in the development of local services.

Isolation hospital provision was a common area for local authority coordination: epidemics were unreliable, on the wane, and difficult to plan for, and therefore sharing hospital space with other councils was one way for smaller authorities in particular to reduce costs while ensuring adequate coverage for their population. As we found for Barnsley, such enforced co-operation between municipalities could bring its own problems, and the potentially problematic nature of forging and maintaining good relationships between councils is illustrated also in West Hartlepool.

As early as 1919 West Hartlepool had accepted the recommendation of the Local Government Board to provide hospital accommodation for infectious cases, instead of using the inadequate facilities of the Port

Authority.[48] Owing to a combination of legal problems and the Geddes cuts, no progress had been made by 1925 when the Ministry suggested the local authorities of the area combine to provide a joint isolation hospital.[49] However, the events of the following months revealed the poor relationship between West Hartlepool, Hartlepool and the Port Authority, and position the Town Clerk as central to the difficulties. The negotiations provide an illuminating example of the impact of petty local rivalries on health service development.

The three authorities had agreed early in 1926 to bring in an expert, the MOH of Leeds, Dr Jervis, to make an assessment of the problems with the Port's hospital and on the suitability of any future site.[50] Problems arose when West Hartlepool's MOH started his correspondence with Dr Jervis, which offended the chief official of the port authority, Mr Bunting, who felt sidelined as a result. West Hartlepool's Town Clerk, H. W. Stanton, believing his own authority should retain control of the project, refused to co-operate with Mr Bunting, who in retaliation called a 'secret' meeting excluding West Hartlepool representatives. When West Hartlepool then tried to call its own rival meeting, Hartlepool officials refused to attend, as they felt the Port Authority should be leading the scheme.[51] The bad feeling between the councils remained, with each authority blaming the other, leading West Hartlepool to decide that the best course was to provide its own isolation facilities.[52] By this time, however, the 'business party' on the council was in ascendance, and although an outbreak of enteric fever

48 MOH Annual Report, West Hartlepool, 1918, p. 31. The borough had actually purchased some land for an infectious diseases hospital in Brierton Lane in 1903, but had never built on it; 'West Hartlepool Council Proposals,' *Northern Daily Mail*, 4 June 1919. For a perspective on the role and development of port authorities in relation to Liverpool, see S. Sheard, 'Mixed Motives: Improving the Health of Seamen in Liverpool 1875–1939', <http://phoenixtn.net/publication/evora/papersOriginal/MixedMotivesHealthofSeamen.doc>, accessed 9 March 2010.

49 Teesside Archives CB/WH/C2/177, West Hartlepool Health Committee Minutes, 13 May, 26 August and 28 October 1925.

50 Ibid. 24 February 1926.

51 Ibid. 24 February 1926.

52 Ibid. 17 March 1926.

in 1929 helped to focus the minds of councillors, a hospital solely servicing West Hartlepool's population was not finally opened until the spring of 1933.[53]

If relations with outside local authorities and the Ministry of Health could retard service provision, this did not mean that relations between the different health providers within the West Hartlepool district were any easier. Although the council part-controlled the voluntary Cameron Hospital through representatives on its Board, this did not translate into easy co-operation, while throughout the period the municipality was on consistently poor terms with the Hartlepools Hospital, the other voluntary hospital of the town. The poor relationship between the three bodies played a major role in the non-appropriation of West Hartlepool's PAI, Howbeck.

Howbeck Infirmary and ex-workhouse was located a mile and a half to the north of town and was also a home for mentally deficient patients, as well as having a number of beds allocated for VD cases sent from the town clinic.[54] There had been developments in the medical services of the infirmary in the late 1920s, but their effectiveness was hampered by the inevitable lack of municipal investment. Following the passing of the 1929 Local Government Act and after having consulted local GPs the MOH, Dr McKeggie, constructed two different schemes for the future of Howbeck infirmary and for cooperation with the voluntary hospitals. The basis of both schemes was the presumption that sufficient hospital accommodation in the town existed, but that it was poorly organised: 'In the event of the lunatics being removed from the hospital, the Council would have a surplus number of beds, which could be used either to cope with the overflow of patients awaiting admission to other general hospitals, or for further extension of its present use'.[55]

53 MOH Annual Report, West Hartlepool, 1929, pp. 4–5.

54 TNA MH66/988, Survey Report, West Hartlepool, 47; Teesside Archives CB/WH/C2/176 and CB/WH/C2/178, West Hartlepool Health Committee Minutes, 28 May 1919 and 25 April 1928.

55 Teesside Archives CB/WH/C2/180, West Hartlepool Health Committee Minutes, 16 April 1930, Report of the MOH on Howbeck Infirmary Submitted to the Committee.

McKeggie's overall aim was that an appropriated Howbeck should be used as a 'clearing station, or central hospital, to be utilised in conjunction with the other two hospitals'.[56] He personally favoured the refurbishment of Howbeck and an increase in resident and consultative staff.[57] In this plan a subscription scheme was to be run via certain clubs, societies and works, to allow cases to be treated for a fixed sum, with non-contributors being assessed according to their means. However, the local branch of the BMA was unanimous in its support for a second scheme which would entail no extra building, in which staff at Howbeck remained the same except for one more Resident Medical Officer and certain specialist appointments.[58]

It is certainly the case that within the council there were interest groups and individuals – notably the Public Assistance Committee and its chair, Alderman Hyde – who were resistant to appropriation in any form and who did their best to slow down change. It was not until 1936 when Labour gained control of the council that the question of improving Howbeck really entered on to the council's agenda. However, it is equally clear that the poor relationship with and between the voluntary hospitals was also a major factor in the non-appropriation of, and continued lack of investment in, the infirmary, and consequent ongoing lack of organised hospital services generally in the town. In the discussions over the future of the hospital, and whether it should be improved, or a new hospital built, it became clear that the voluntary hospitals were unwilling to co-operate in any new scheme. At a meeting between council representatives and the Ministry it transpired

56 Ibid. West Hartlepool Health Committee Minutes, 21 April 1931.

57 In this scheme the hospital was to have had around 400 beds and the mental deficiency colony 230 beds. These would be placed under the care of a resident medical superintendent (salary £700) and two resident assistants (salary £200). This would entail building a kitchen, the superintendent's house and providing extra accommodation for the assistants.

58 TNA MH66/990, Survey Appendices, West Hartlepool, Letter From MOH Dr McKeggie to the Members of the Health Committee, 24 November 1930. For an insight into the attitudes interwar GPs, the section of the medical profession especially active in local BMA branches, see A. Digby and N. Bosanquet, 'Doctors and Patients in an Era of National Health Insurance and Private Practice, 1913–1938', *Economic History Review*, 41:1 (1988).

that the council had not formally asked the Cameron for its views on the proposal, nor approached Hartlepools Hospital to see if they would join in a joint scheme. The council deputation explained this by saying that 'there was considerable local feeling which hindered cooperation between West Hartlepool and Hartlepool, and they were extremely doubtful whether the Hartlepools hospital would agree to take part in any scheme involving cooperation with the hospitals in West Hartlepool'.[59]

A visit to the town in 1939 by a Ministry inspector, Dr Maitland, to assess the need for a new hospital as opposed to improving Howbeck was revealing of the position of the voluntary hospitals. Hartlepools Hospital (situated in West Hartlepool County Borough) was by far the largest, with ninety-five beds, and strong links with the miners' associations, and was in a strong financial position owing to 'the flourishing work people's contributory scheme.'[60] Representatives for the Hospital thought that the only area in which there was likely to be cooperation with the other hospitals was pathology, which was only slightly developed in all three institutions anyway. They thought that any fuller cooperation was 'precluded by the difficulties of unifying the practices of a hospital dependent on a contributory scheme, another voluntary institution without such a scheme and one publicly owned.'[61] These representatives did not attend the conference to which they had been invited by council to meet representatives from the Ministry of Health and the Cameron Hospital. Dr Maitland observed that he had 'little doubt that neither the Board nor the medical staff have any intention of agreeing to any substantial alterations in practice, to secure cooperation ... There will be cooperation no doubt so long as they can continue to carry on all the services that they want'.[62]

59 TNA MH66/995, Resurvey Correspondence, West Hartlepool, Resume of Meeting Held Between West Hartlepool County Borough Officials and Ministry of Health, 30 January 1939.

60 Ibid. Report on Visit to Investigate Alternative Accommodation for Extending General Hospital Accommodation in West Hartlepool, Dr Maitland, 6 June 1939.

61 Ibid.

62 Ibid.

So, while we stress the importance of understanding the role of councillors in inhibiting health service developments through their unwillingness to spend, we have also shown in this section how it is crucial to set this in the context of the actions of other health providers in the borough. Even when the council made efforts towards improving their hospital provision – both isolation and general – the examples we have used have shown how both other local authorities and voluntary hospitals could be obstructive. This resulted in painfully slow progress, resulting in either no improvements or glacially creeping developments.

However, this did not always have to be the case, and in this final part of the chapter we show an example of improvements to a service through the development of synergistic relations with other health care providers. This was the development of the municipal antenatal and maternity services, which we have seen failed to attract further investment after the initial post-World War One period of expansion. Its continued development was instead based on improved relationships with the medical practitioners of the town. In 1925 the MOH stated how:

> On its initiation several years ago there was no coordination between the local [authority's health visitor service] and the doctors, and the latter rather resented the idea of Corporation nurses 'poking their noses' into cases in their practice. That feeling has now disappeared. The procedure was adopted five years ago of stamping on the birth notification forms 'Do you wish a Health Visitor to visit this case – Yes or No'. At first a negative answer was returned in the great majority of cases. When, however, it was realised that we weren't out to interfere but rather to help there seemed to be a complete change over.[63]

This take-up was further improved by the introduction of a council maternity insurance scheme in 1928. This was designed to get round the rising incidence of fees borne by the council when a doctor was called to attend a birth in an emergency, which could not be recouped from the patient.[64]

63 MOH Annual Report, West Hartlepool, 1925, p. 43.

64 Councils were bound to follow this procedure under the 1918 Maternity and Child Welfare Act. See, for example, 'Poor Patients', *Northern Daily Mail*, 7 February 1923, and West Hartlepool MOH Annual Report, 1928, p. 20.

It was actually prompted by a desire to save money rather than a wish to improve the maternity service for women, but in fact the new scheme did both. A contribution of five shillings covered a woman for emergency health care during confinement and afterwards. Where women were not insured and called in a doctor, the council tried to 'extract the full fee, [and sent] them a note to the effect that if they had been insured it would not have been necessary to send them an account'.[65] Six months into the scheme, the Borough Treasurer and the MOH calculated that the scheme had saved the council roughly 20 per cent on what the maternity services had cost the previous financial year. The MOH believed that the scheme was 'an advantageous one', as it provided 'a source of comfort for the mother', and for the midwife, who now knew she would not be blamed for calling in a doctor if anything went wrong. However, he acknowledged that the 'weakness in the scheme is that the patient having paid her premium insists on the midwife calling for the doctor although the necessity has not arisen'. There was also the problem that it was women who had had complications in the past who were more likely to take out insurance, meaning the council were 'insuring bad cases'.[66]

Within the Public Health Committee the enthusiasm felt for the scheme in its early years waned as the Borough Treasurer's returns increasingly showed that it was becoming less and less cost effective, notwithstanding its popularity amongst the town's women, and the approval it received from the Ministry of Health.[67] By 1932 the MOH was protesting that the council had arrears going back seven years 'and in a large number of cases there is no hope of recovery and nothing has been collected for a

65 MOH Annual Report, West Hartlepool, 1929, p. 27.

66 MOH Annual Report, West Hartlepool, 1928, pp. 20–1. The council was empowered to do this under the Midwives' and Maternity Homes Act, 1926. Of the 118 women who took out insurance and were confined during the first six months of the scheme, fifty-one cases had medical treatment at a cost of £60. 8s. in doctor's fees, for which the council received £29. 10s. in premiums. Therefore the cost to the council for each case treated was 12s. 1d., compared to 17s. under the old system.

67 TNA MH66/988, Survey Report, West Hartlepool, 23.

considerable time'.[68] The council was more optimistic about the chances of recovering the payments, but it is clear that many of the people involved were (in the Town Clerk's words) 'quite unable to pay the claims made against them'.[69] It is typical of the council at this time that the success of the scheme was measured in sterling rather than in terms of the benefits to the townswomen's health, although they may also have had legal obligations to pursue defaulters.

The third key development in the town's maternity service in these years was the result of a resolution on antenatal care passed by the local branch of the BMA in 1931. This appears to have stemmed from their desire to prevent the municipal health department from encroaching into what they saw as their territory. The BMA resolved that all pregnant women coming to the attention of the MOH should in future be referred to private practitioners.[70] A doctor was to be nominated by the patient to attend her confinement in cases of emergency, 'with a view to those doctors being given an opportunity of doing the necessary antenatal examinations', at no charge to the council. Given the mindset of the majority of the council, and their dislike of employing more health staff than necessary, it is unsurprising that the Public Health Committee gave the proposal their enthusiastic backing.[71] Co-operation was cheerfully adopted in this case, but again, the significance of financial savings was paramount.

These examples show that significant extensions to the town's maternity services could take place in the context of an economising council concerned with reducing expenditure rather than expanding service provision. This is not to claim that the health services during the reign of the business party were not underfunded and patchy – as the Ministry of Health survey of the towns services made it clear that they were both these

68 The council employed a collector, Mr Pearson, who received a 20 per cent commission on each debt he recovered.

69 Teesside Archives CB/WH/C2/182, West Hartlepool Health Committee Minutes, 28 May 1934. See also CB/WH/C2/181, West Hartlepool Health Committee Minutes, 25 April 1932 for the more optimistic view on recovering outstanding fees.

70 On the attitudes of GPs, see Digby and Bosanquet, 'Doctors and Patients'.

71 Teesside Archives CB/WH/C2/181, West Hartlepool Health Committee Minutes, 22 June 1931.

things – but that we must be wary of automatically equating reductions in council spending with the contraction of services. Where other healthcare providers could be called upon to bear the cost of an improved service, the council was much more likely to think about co-operating.

Conclusions

Our exploration of the West Hartlepool case study has revealed how the town was in some ways atypical of its geographical context: its industry was more diversified; unemployment, while high, was lower than surrounding towns; Labour was slow to make gains on the council and had weak links with local trade unions; and the 'business party' that dominated municipal politics for the central years of the interwar period ensured that efforts towards slum clearance and the improvement of the lives of the poor attempted elsewhere were slow to take root in the town. Its rateable value was low, but it is also clear that the council consciously chose to prioritise reductions in the amount of rate set in the pound at a time when other poorly off boroughs, such as Barnsley, were making increases. This extreme reluctance to increase outlay resulted in below-average levels of investment in the health services throughout the interwar period.

To an extent the characteristics of West Hartlepool which drove its selection as a low Labour, low spending borough have been reinforced by the qualitative archival evidence. For the central decade of the period, 1926–1936, the council had far lower than average Labour representation and spent far under the County Borough average on municipal health services to the extent that the 1929 Local Government Act actually coincidence with a reduction in outlay. This ensured that at the time of the first Ministry of Health survey in 1931 the inspector found flaws and limitations in every aspect of provision, and that an acrimonious relationship developed between the council and the Ministry which became increasingly frustrated by the recalcitrant attitude of councillors. In this the council was very different from our other case study boroughs, which all to one extent or another attempted to engage with suggestions put forward by the Ministry, even if they too were sometimes slow in acting.

Yet in this chapter we have also shown the importance of going beyond the quantitative aggregate material, revealing that before 1922 and after 1936 we can in fact chart different patterns of spending and attitudes towards service expansion. Using the MCW services and TB provision as examples it is clear that West Hartlepool presented a more complex picture than first suggested. While the period of expansion after 1936 can be strongly linked to national – and especially local – economic recovery, plus Labour taking over the council in the town, and so at least in part confirming our hypothesis of the importance of politics in the provision of municipal services, the rise in spending in the period before 1922 is less easily explained. Expansion before the Geddes cuts can perhaps be best understood as part of a national context of a new health ministry, the granting of extensive powers to County Borough councils, and an absence of anti-spend councillors in the town. As the drive to improvements brought about by these novelties lost momentum, and the business party gained it, investment slowed right down. The example of the maternity insurance scheme, however, reveals how improvements in services could still take place even in the context of a parsimonious council intent on saving money.

As well as pointing to the need to pay close attention to change over time, the material from West Hartlepool – in common with Newport – also suggests how important it is to take account of the other bodies providing health services in the borough. An examination of the council's relationship with other local authorities and voluntary hospitals shows how very often the parochial and narrow interests of other parties, as much as the council's own unwillingness to spend, resulted in delays, blind alleys and stagnation. However, a new inclination to work with other councils and the voluntary hospital after 1936 does suggest that the Labour council brought with it a changed attitude to co-operation as much as a different approach to spending, as shown in their own statements on the health services. West Hartlepool may well have been a poor 'stinter', but council decisions did not exist in isolation: the complex web of voluntary hospitals, shared services and GPs ensured its decisions were entangled in a wealth of local concerns and jealousies that were a significant feature of interwar health care provision.

CHAPTER EIGHT

Conclusions

As we set out in Chapter One, we have aimed in this book to examine municipal medicine in a wider sense than generally considered previously. At the risk of some oversimplification, most previous studies have taken a somewhat reductionist approach, focusing on the provision of healthcare services – the 'medical' – but with less grounding in the politics of what was, after all, a political system. We argue that many studies view municipal medicine through a centralist lens, and have attempted to examine a local political system without the local decision making context. We have aimed to draw the two aspects of local provision together, placing the 'municipal' back into 'municipal medicine'.

We also claim that considerations of municipal healthcare have not been nuanced enough; particularly in terms of their geographical scope, their scale and the way that they changed over even the relatively short timeframe of the interwar period. While there has been some focus on different parts of the municipal medical sector and of municipal medicine in different localities, there has not been a comprehensive treatment of the sector in Britain since the studies of Wilson.[1]

However, it is important to examine municipal medicine for five main reasons. First, it was an essential, but relatively neglected, part of health care before the NHS, being the quantitative backbone of the hospital 'system' in terms of number of institutions, expenditure, staffing, beds, and patients treated, as well as being the principal provider of services such as MCW. During the interwar period – the zenith of municipal medicine[2] – the

1 N. Wilson, *Public Health Services* (London, 1938); N. Wilson, *Municipal Health Services* (London, 1946).

2 J. Pickstone, *Medicine and Industrial Society. A History of Hospital Development in Manchester and its Region, 1752–1946* (Manchester, 1985), 6.

sector was an 'expanding service'[3] and one which, in its own terms, enjoyed some success in the sense of providing an improving service for its residents. Second, the municipal structure itself has great significance because it was the accepted model for healthcare right up to the inception of the NHS after the Second World War. Indeed, Bevan's move to a nationalised model surprised many contemporaries of all political persuasions, who expected and desired a municipalisation of the health service. Third concerns an important context for future policy: there have been many claims since 1948 that the NHS suffers from a 'democratic deficit', that nationalisation was a great mistake, that it is time to reassess the Bevan-Morrison Cabinet debate, and that some measure of democratisation and municipalisation should be considered.[4] In this sense, an examination of municipal medicine provides a potential basis for 'counterfactual' analysis – how might this 'road not taken' throw some light on future policy options? Fourth, municipal medicine is an important, though overlooked, element in the 'cradle to grave' local welfare state before 1945, which was recognised at the time. This leads to our title – cradle to grave – a phrase normally associated with the Beveridge model of the 'welfare state.' Fifth, the study aims to provide a more nuanced picture in a broader context, leading to a more balanced portrayal of an era in health care provision often characterised as backward or stagnant. In particular, it provides a wider and alternative focus of examination of a local welfare state examined through a localist rather than a centralist lens.[5]

The accounts that have dealt with the pre-NHS health services have offered varied interpretations of its range and quality, and feature both optimistic and pessimistic conclusions. However, in a wider view, elements of both the optimistic and pessimistic views are correct in two broad senses. First, localism led to great geographical variation, meaning that both opti-

3 M. Powell, 'An Expanding Service: Municipal Acute Medicine in the 1930s', *Twentieth Century British History*, 8:3 (1997).

4 See Chapter One for an overview of these accounts and debates.

5 Page, 'Localism and Centralism'; Ibid. 'The Value'; D. Ashford, *The Emergence of Welfare States* (Oxford, 1986); Powell, 'In What Sense'; Powell and Boyne, 'The Spatial Strategy'.

mistic and pessimistic accounts can coexist. Second, the level of optimism depends on the comparative template and what, given the political and macro- and micro-economic circumstances of the time, could be regarded as 'reasonable' or 'realistic' degrees of progress (assuming, of course, that volume of resources is a proxy for quality, which – as we showed in our case studies – was not necessarily the case). We claim that the historiography suffers from a range of problems, which include a number of misleading claims and assertions without evidence. In particular, much of the literature is limited as it takes an aggregate rather than a disaggregate view, focuses on a static rather than a dynamic picture, and, as already noted, does not place municipal medicine within a wider localist political system. From a localist point of view, variation that results from political choice, for example, is very different from economic constraint. In other words, it is important to differentiate situations where local authorities chose not to spend from those where they were unable to spend.

We began our analysis at a national level in Chapter Two, where we examined expenditure by the local authorities with the greatest range of healthcare responsibilities, the County Boroughs. This analysis was carried out via three perspectives: over time, over space and between healthcare sectors. We found that the dichotomy between 'spenders' and 'stinters' posited by Hicks and Hicks is too simplistic a scheme, as it misses the dynamic picture of differential growth and differential spending priorities.[6] In other words, a stinter on mental hospitals may be a spender on MCW, and a stinter in 1922 may be a spender in 1936. Nor does a crude north-south explain expenditure levels: instead our analysis showed that there was considerable variation within every region examined. The large south-east region, for example, contained the second highest ranking borough in terms of overall expenditure – West Ham – alongside the second lowest – Portsmouth. Attention was also drawn to the impact of the historiographically neglected 1929 Local Government Act, which abolished

6 J. R. Hicks and U. K. Hicks, 'Standards of Local Expenditure. A Problem of the Inequality of Incomes', *Occasional Papers*, National Institute of Economic and Social Research (Cambridge, 1943).

the Poor Law Unions, brought their functions into the remit of the local authorities, and made provision for their medical institutions to be 'appropriated' to Public Health functions as well as changing the structure of local authority grants.

In Chapter Three we began to drill down to find some explanations for these differing patterns, and in particular, the reasons behind their different paths of development. Using the 1930s Ministry of Health surveys of individual boroughs' medical services, we argued that the development of health services depended on an assortment of local factors. These ranged from the size of the rate base, local antagonisms, commitments to other priorities, perceived poverty, relations with the voluntary sector, political composition and style of the council, the influence of individuals like the MOH and the council Treasurer, relations with other local and central authorities, and a tendency to extravagance or apathy, among others. The Ministry's health surveys also strongly suggest that general hospitals after the 1929 Local Government Act followed a different path from the other health services. The Ministry of Health inspectors called upon a similar range of factors affecting progress as those used for municipal health services more generally, but it is clear that some were particularly charged in this arena. In particular, expense, relations between different council committees, voluntary bodies and local authority neighbours, and attitudes to the buildings themselves could play a large part. We also criticised a focus on appropriation as an event rather than a process, arguing that it is important to examine what happened to the general hospitals after the appropriation decision – or lack thereof. We also highlighted the significance of more practical factors, most notably the nature of the inheritance from the Poor Law Guardians in 1930 and the ease with which this could be modernised or developed for acute medical and surgical care. Finally, we turned to correlation and regression analysis of the factors affecting spending levels. This found a clear tendency for Labour-dominated boroughs to spend more on average, and that the difference became more pronounced over the period. As high Labour areas also tended to have low rateable values, the political and economic factors promoting high spending tended to be in conflict, however, but when the political factor was examined – ceteris paribus– in regression terms, its effect tended to strengthen. These findings were used to introduce the need for detailed local-level studies to probe these tensions and impetuses further. These were identified on the basis of their levels of Labour representation on the council, and their wealth. As there were few rich, Labour and poor non-Labour areas, we selected areas that scored high or low in *relative* terms: Barnsley (poor/ high Labour); Eastbourne (wealthy/ low Labour); Newport (wealthy/ high Labour); West Hartlepool (poor; low Labour).

The second part of the book (Chapters Four to Seven) developed these detailed case studies of municipal healthcare services. Considered together, they highlight the range of factors which affected healthcare provision, illustrating many of the themes discussed in the earlier chapters. Barnsley, for example, shows the influence of Labour politics on spending decisions, but also highlights how far Labour was a locally constructed identity. In this borough it was heavily influenced by miners' organisations and trade unions, and was well organised and combative. Here, it did help effect high spending levels despite a poor rate base and severe depression. Labour councillors consistently pressed for reform on the areas of MCW and hospital services in particular. It was the only one of our four case studies to appropriate its transferred institution.

The examination of Eastbourne County Borough showed a completely different type of town. Most obviously, it was much wealthier than Barnsley, with a large proportion of retired residents, and a significant pull for visitors because of its status as a seaside resort. It also had low levels of Labour representation throughout the period. Nonetheless, it spent at very high levels on municipal health, largely because of its wealth, coupled with a long-held pride in its standards of health. The long-serving and forceful MOH, William Willoughby, was another major force for action. The voluntary sector had a prominent profile in this town, but the particular preference for supporting and developing institutions was continued into the municipal arena as well. The depth of civic pride in the Eastbourne was seen in a commitment to flagship institutions for health care, like the infectious disease and TB hospitals, and also the voluntary institution, the Princess Alice. This position was not upheld throughout the period, however, and in its latter years there was a significant tendency to retrenchment and economy. Indeed, by the second half of our period, the borough was being outstripped by Barnsley in expenditure terms. This again points to the need to unpick seemingly attractive labels at a more micro level: Eastbourne's association with 'spending' was converted into a tendency to 'stinting' by the second half of the period.

Our rich/ high Labour borough of Newport illustrated localism in another form; namely in its relationship with the distinctive provider of TB services in Wales, the Welsh National Memorial Association. This case study also demonstrates the local flavour of Labour politics: it lacked strong leaders, and its forcefulness and style of governance was very different from the party in Barnsley. Instead, the voluntary sector played a much larger part in setting the remit of the municipal health services. Among all our case studies, Newport was the town which relied most heavily on voluntary agencies to fulfil the council's various health service obligations. Unlike our other three towns, it did not have a municipal maternity home, for example, relying initially on a voluntary aided home, and later on, the private sector. This presents a challenge to the view that Labour sought out its own projects; in Newport the party was sympathetic to the prominent role of the voluntary sector (as we saw also in the case of the voluntary hospital in Barnsley). In Newport, however, Labour involvement was not in itself enough to prompt above-average levels of expenditure on health.

Our final case study, West Hartlepool, revealed the struggles between centre and local authorities in action. This town had neither of the key factors predisposing high expenditure: it was quite a poorly off borough and Labour had little sway on its council. Our investigation found that it was also almost consistently opposed to schemes which would bring greater levels of investment. This was partly due to sensitivity to the rate burden and partly a reflection of priorities in other areas, but it also reflects a lack of strong direction in the health field. Municipal politics were dominated to varying degrees across the whole period by 'business-minded' independents, and the Ministry of Health in the early 1930s recorded a 'stupid and ... obstinate resistance of a powerful section of the Council' to health service development at this time.[7] However, from November

7 TNA MH66/993, Resurvey Report, West Hartlepool, 5. See Chapter Seven for more on this comment.

1936 Labour was able to construct a working majority on the council, and although we lack the financial statistics to quantify the change in spending that resulted from this political shift, this was accompanied by an upsurge in activity within the council's health services, most notably in MCW, and TB services. The need for micro-level study of broad-brush characterisations is again highlighted.

Explaining Municipal Medicine

This book has thus taken a twofold approach to investment in municipal medicine. First, we have sought to map out patterns of expenditure variously at geographic, temporal and sectoral levels. Second, we have used qualitative national data, and then a range of detailed local information in four micro-historical studies to try to explain the factors which shaped the national patterns. We have argued that explaining the development of municipal medicine requires the examination of a complex web of interacting factors, and that these interactions varied in significance according to individual sectors. This is especially true when considering general hospitals.

The strongest explanations for the patterns we uncover come from issues where the quantitative expenditure analysis and the case study archival evidence suggest similar conclusions. It is clear that wealth in the form of local rateable value was a major factor shaping health care expenditure. In particular, many so-called 'stinters' had limited financial resources, while some 'spenders' had a more expansive rate base. Wealth was, however, not *necessarily* related to high expenditure on health, since the latter also involved a decision on how high to set taxes. A poor borough could thus raise enough money to support greater investment if they were prepared to set a high rate in the pound (as did Barnsley). As we showed in Chapter Two rateable value per head was correlated with public health expenditure per head at only 0.441 in 1922, and fell thereafter. After 1930 the correlation almost disappeared, suggesting that the new block grant brought in 1929 was levelling the playing field across boroughs with different rateable values.[8] This contrasts with findings for the Edwardian period which show much higher levels of correlation.[9] Either health services were less well correlated with wealth than other aspects of rate expenditure, or the relationship had declined significantly, on a national basis at least, by the interwar period. By this time some rich boroughs were spending at a comparatively low(er) level (as we found for Eastbourne by the second half of the period), while some poorer ones were willing to dig deep in order to spend highly (as in Barnsley).

Our analysis has also highlighted, however, that these broad trends were not necessarily applicable across the whole range of municipal health services, and that some boroughs prioritised one or two services while spending at a lower level on others – regardless of their rateable value. These trends were clearly observed in our case studies, where perceived need, local tradition, and the interests of individuals meant that some services attracted particular investment. The 'stinting' borough of West Hartlepool, for example, did invest at something close to the national average on mental deficiency, and MCW, in the early years of the period, at least, while spending at much lower levels on other health services. This conclusion holds true at an even more detailed level: for example, expenditure on TB services in Eastbourne went disproportionately into the dispensary rather than into X-rays, while within MCW schemes the provision of free milk was prominent.

8 J. P. Bradbury, 'The 1929 Local Government Act: The Formulation and Implementation of Poor Law (Health Care) and Exchequer Grants Reform for England and Wales (Outside London)', PhD thesis, University of Bristol, 1991, states that the change in the grant system under the 1929 Act did not adversely affect expenditure on services which had previously been aided by the percentage grants. He does however provide evidence of County Boroughs where the block grant 'confirmed reactionary attitudes' (302), or was used 'to arrest even existing development' (305). The poorer boroughs were probably the most adversely affected, especially given the national drive for economy, which prompted many of them to use the grant to reduce pressure on the local rates.

9 B. T. Preston, 'Rich Town, Poor Town: The Distribution of Rate-Borne Spending Levels in the Edwardian City System', *Transactions of the Institute of British Geographers*, New Series, 10 (1985).

Our analysis has also highlighted the separate range of inter-related factors which affected the appropriation and development of general hospitals compared with the other services. At the most basic level, we have argued that appropriation did not follow the path of the other sectors as it depended most crucially on whether a suitable institution was inherited from the Poor Law Guardians after the 1929 Local Government Act. Appropriation was debated in all four of our case study towns, but only Barnsley ultimately went ahead with this course of action. The reasons given by the other case study towns illustrate a range of other factors at play, from anxiety about raised costs, antagonisms between committees on the council, and the nature of relations with the voluntary sector and other local municipal authorities. Some of these debates also reveal the nature of 'hierarchical regionalism', which were to inform the post-war approach of Aneurin Bevan – although in several cases we see tensions between different types of local authority rather than co-operation.[10] Nonetheless, the negotiations between our case study councils and other 'lesser' local authorities, are revealing of attitudes to specialisation and the roles of different towns in a local area. This particularly affected the development of hospital provision; a further reminder that in economic terms a developed municipal hospital sector was sometimes beyond the resources of smaller boroughs. This might be exacerbated by a local voluntary hospital with a much wider catchment area, especially for boroughs situated near a large town with an attractive hospital.

Our study has also allowed us to make some advances in understanding the nature of the Labour Party's influence on spending. Regression analysis pointed to a clear and growing relationship between local party seats held, and high levels of expenditure. However, it remains clear that the Labour Party had its greatest early successes in places with relatively poor levels of resources, and poor socio-economic indicators of health and well-being. The case studies have been particularly revealing for understanding how these apparently competing factors were played out. In particular,

10 D. M. Fox, *Health Policies, Health Politics: The British and American Experience, 1911–1965* (Princeton, 1986).

they have underlined the need to build up a picture of the Labour Party which is locally specific. Barnsley and Newport both had high levels of Labour representation, for example, but the parties had entirely different characters. The strength of the party could also be considerably restrained by other local coalitions and interests; as we saw in the case of the Welsh National Memorial Association in Newport, for example. Often, strong-minded individuals could have more influence than political parties, like the MOH, Dr Willoughby, in Eastbourne, or the miners' leader, Herbert Smith, in Barnsley.

Conclusion: Municipalising Municipal Medicine

We will use this final section to highlight a few broad conclusions and reflections. First, we have presented a more nuanced picture of municipal medicine compared with much of the historiography. It is important to focus on a disaggregate analysis that explores variations over time, space and sector. It follows that there is no simple pattern of 'spenders' and 'stinters'.

Second, our conclusions tend to be more positive than much of the previous historiography, especially in terms of their assessment of local agency. Although provision in some areas was clearly very poor, that in others was relatively good and improving. We therefore highlight room for optimism about the vibrancy of localism, if not always its efficacy.

Third, explanations are complex. Single factors such as economic determinism are not sufficient. Although explanations are multidimensional, we have given more weight to political *choice*. It is important to differentiate this from party colour *per se*. It is clear that local authorities made their own expenditure decisions– but not always in circumstances of their own choosing.

Finally, we have argued that much analysis has been conducted through a centralist rather than a localist lens, which offers an incomplete picture for this period of high municipalism. Rodney Lowe and Neil Rollings suggest that historians, unlike political scientists, have tended to accept the 'Westminster narrative.'[11] This ignores the importance of local government as a welfare state. We argued in Chapter One that there are clear differences between national and local welfare states. However, many commentators tend implicitly to evaluate the local welfare state of municipal medicine in the interwar period on 'national' criteria, ignoring any positive achievements of those in the 'local' arena. In a similar sense, commentators have taken the side of Bevan rather than Morrison in the Cabinet debate of 1945 on the future of the health services. However, as we saw in Chapter One, some writers consider that nationalisation was a great blow to local government; was Labour's great mistake; and feel that the debate should be revisited. We will end with some brief reflection on how this question relates to the lessons learned from our study.

Rudolph Klein has pointed to a clear ideological split between Bevan and Morrison, not in party terms but in terms of perceived values. On the one hand are Morrison's political values: the emphasis on local government as a school of political education and active citizenship, with considerations of efficiency and administrative rationality coming a poor second. On the other hand, is Bevan's stress on a different set of values: those of paternalistic rationalism and uniformity of provision. He argued that the NHS represented a clash of values. The 1948 Bevan model represented the victory of rationality, efficiency and equity: it was designed to be the instrument of national policies for delivering health care in a rational, efficient and fair way across the country. But the case for local government was based on a view of the world anchored in the values of localism: a view which stressed responsiveness rather than efficiency, differentiation rather than uniformity, self-government rather than national equity.[12]

11 R. Lowe and N. Rollings, 'Modernising Britain, 1957–64: A Classic Case of Centralisation and Fragmentation?' in R. A. W. Rhodes, ed., *Transforming British Government,* i: *Changing Institutions* (London, 2000), 99.

12 Klein, *The New Politics*, 15, 22.

This narrative fits with Bevan's pursuit of power from Tredegar Urban District Council, to Monmouthshire County Council, to Westminster. Foot recounts that this began when Nye was a young boy:

> 'Very important man. That's Councillor Jackson' his father had said to him. 'What's the Council?' he asked. 'Very important place indeed and they are very powerful men' his father had replied. 'When I got older I said to myself; the place to get to is the Council. That's where the power is. So I worked very hard and, in association with my fellows, when I was about twenty years of age, I got on the Council. I discovered when I got there that the power had been there, but it had just gone. So I made some enquiries, being an earnest student of social affairs, and I learned that the power had slipped down to the County Council. That was where it was and where it had gone to. So I worked very hard again and I got there and it had gone from there too.'[13]

This was clearly a partial and probably self-serving, even teleological, view. While Bevan's pursuit of power took him to Westminster, medical historians should not follow him in their pursuit of municipal medicine. In the interwar period, much power still remained at local level, and it is here that the pursuit should be focused. There was nothing 'inevitable' about the creation of a centralised NHS just as there was nothing 'inevitable' about Bevan's journey from pithead to Parliament. Municipal medicine in interwar England and Wales needs to be seen and understood in its own terms – nuanced and highly differentiated, but not necessarily a failing system which cried out for replacement by a 'top down' version of socialised healthcare.

13 M. Foot, *Aneurin Bevan. A Biography* i: *1897–1945* (London, 1966), 71–2.

Bibliography

Primary Sources

Official Papers

Annual Reports of the Chief Medical Officer, 1919–35
Annual Reports of the Ministry of Health, 1919–39
Census of England and Wales, 1921, 1931.
Local Government Board, Forty-Eighth Annual Report 1919, Cmd. 462, vi.
Local Government During the Period of Reconstruction, 1944–5, Cmnd 6579, x.
Medical Officer of Health, Annual Reports, Barnsley, Eastbourne, Newport, West Hartlepool, 1919–39.
Society of Medical Officers of Health, *The White Paper on a National Health Service* (London, 1944).
Ministry of Health, *A National Health Service*, Cmnd. 6502 (London: HMSO, 1944).
Ministry of Health, Nuffield Provincial Hospital Trust Hospital Survey (London, 1945–6).
Hansard, *Parliamentary Debates.*
Reports of the Registrar General, 1931–5.
Report of the Committee of Inquiry in the Anti-Tuberculosis Service in Wales and Monmouthshire (London, 1939).
Report on Maternal Mortality in Wales, 1937, Cmd. 5423, xi.

Political and Economic Planning

The Hospital System. Planning Broadsheet, 84 (London, 1934).
The Hospital System (London, 1936).
Report on the British Health Services (London, 1937).
Report on the British Social Services (London, 1937).
Medical Care for Citizens, Planning Broadsheet 222 (London, 1944).

The National Archives (TNA)

CAB/3, The Future of the Hospital services, Cabinet Papers, 1945.

Ministry of Health Records

TNA MH55/1198, Anti-tuberculosis committee for Wales.
TNA MH61/30, Commissioners for the Special Areas.

MH66 Ministry of Health, Local Government Act 1929 Public Health Survey, 1930–43
/991, Survey Correspondence, West Hartlepool.
/420, Survey Report, Barnsley, Appendices.
/421, Survey Report, Barnsley.
/454, Survey Report, Blackpool.
/459, Survey Report, Bolton.
/473, Survey Report, Bournemouth.
/476, Survey Correspondence, Bournemouth.
/487, Survey Report, Bristol.
/507, Resurvey Correspondence, Burton-on-Trent.
/571, Survey Report, Darlington.
/577, Survey Report, Derby.
/584, Survey Report, Doncaster.
/596, Survey Correspondence, Eastbourne.
/625, Survey Report, Gloucester.
/665, Survey Report, Hastings.
/718, Survey Report, Lincoln.
/721, Survey Report, Liverpool.
/898, Survey Report, Stockport.
/988, Survey Report, West Hartlepool.
/990, Survey Appendices, West Hartlepool
/991, Survey Correspondence, West Hartlepool.
/993, Resurvey Report, West Hartlepool.
/995, Resurvey Correspondence, West Hartlepool.
/1066, Survey Report, Barnsley.
/1071, Survey Report, Eastbourne.

MH67/133, Proposed Joint Sanatorium: Conference of Local Authorities: Appendices: Survey of Resources of Area, 1930–1.

MH96, Welsh Board of Health
/61 Newport Blind Services Correspondence, 1925–33
/62, Blind Services in Newport, 1934–8
/387, Survey Report, Newport.
/388, Survey Correspondence, Newport.
/907, Welsh Consultative Council, Maternal Mortality Enquiry, 1922–5.
/1064, Anti-TB Inquiry Report, 1939.
/1099, Newport County Borough Council: Treatment of Tuberculosis Scheme 1920–30
/114–1116, Welsh National Memorial Association, Comparative TB Institution Costs, 1922–39.
/1135, Prevalence of Venereal Disease in Wales, 1918–41.

Barnsley Archives and Local Studies (BALS)

A/1963/G/1, Barnsley Trades Union Council and Labour Party Minute Book, 1916–20.
Minutes of Barnsley County Borough Council 1919–38.

East Sussex Record Office [ESRO]

DE/A5/9–12, Eastbourne Finance and General Purposes Committee Minutes, 1919–45
DE/A7/8–10, Eastbourne Sanitary and Public Health Committee Minutes, 1918–39
DE/A7/13, Eastbourne Maternity and Welfare Committee Minutes, 1918–37,
R/C50/4, St Mary's Institution and Hospital Sub-Committee, May 1931–October 1937

Gwent County Record Office [GCRO]

A110. M26–37, Newport County Borough Council General Council minutes, 1920–30.
A110. M12/1–5, Newport Health Committee, 1920–42.

Swansea Library Archives [SLA]

A.1–7, Records of Newport Constituency Labour Party, Minutes of the Labour Representation Committee, 1918–35.

Teesside Archives

CB/WH/C2/176–84, West Hartlepool Health Committee Minutes, 1919–37.

CB/WH/C2/203, West Hartlepool Joint Consultative Committee on Tuberculosis Minutes, 1919–29.

Wellcome Library for the History and Understanding of Medicine

BMA SA/BMA/F.93, Public Health Files, Contemporary Medical Archives Centre: Completed Questionnaires and Correspondence with Local Authorities and County Boroughs, 1934–5.

Medical Journals

British Medical Journal.
The Lancet.

Newspapers

Barnsley Chronicle.
The Eastbourne Chronicle.
Northern Daily Mail.
Searchlight.
The Newport Searchlight.
South Wales Argus.
South Wales Weekly Argus.
The Times.
Western Mail.

Secondary Sources

'The Health of Eastbourne', *The Medical Officer*, 38 (1927), 247.
Abel-Smith, B., *A History of the Nursing Profession* (London, 1960).
Abel-Smith, B., *The Hospitals 1800–1948* (London, 1964).
Alt, J. E., 'Some Social and Political Correlates of County Borough Expenditures', *British Journal of Political Science*, 1 (1971), 49–62.
Ashford, D., *The Emergence of Welfare States* (Oxford, 1986).
Ayers, G., *England's First State Hospitals 1867–1930* (London, 1971).
Bell, F., and R. Millward, 'Public Health Expenditures and Mortality in England and Wales, 1870–1914', *Continuity and Change*, 13 (1998), 221–49.
Beloff, M., 'The Whitehall Factor: The Role of Higher Civil Service 1919–39', in G. Peele and C. Cook, eds, *The Politics of Reappraisal, 1918–1938* (London, 1975), 209–32.
Blunkett, D., and K. Jackson, *Democracy in Crisis: The Town Halls Respond* (London, 1987).
Boyne, G. A., and M. Powell 'Territorial Justice and Thatcherism' *Environment and Planning C: Government and Policy* 11:1 (1993), 35–53.
Boyne, G. A., *Constraints, choices and public policies* (Greenwich, Conn., 1996).
Bruce, M., *The Coming of the Welfare State* (4th edn, London, 1968).
Bryder, L., 'The King Edward VII Welsh National Association and its Policy Towards Tuberculosis, 1910–48', *Welsh History Review*, 13:2 (1986), 194–215.
Bryder, L., *Below the Magic Mountain: A Social History of Tuberculosis in Twentieth-Century Britain* (Oxford, 1988).
Bulpitt, J. G., *Party Politics in English Local Government* (London, 1967).
Campbell, J., *Nye Bevan and the Mirage of British Socialism* (London, 1987).
Cherry, S., *Medical Services and the Hospitals in Britain, 1860–1939* (Cambridge, 1996).
Cherry, S., 'Regional Comparators in the Funding and Organization of the Voluntary Hospital System, c 1860–1939', in M. Gorsky and S. Sheard, eds, *Financing Medicine: The British Experience Since 1750* (London, 2006), 59–76.
Chester, D. N., *Central and Local Government; Financial and Administrative Relations* (London, 1951).
Clarke, J., *History of the Eastbourne Medical Society, 1883–1983* (Eastbourne, 1983).
Cook, C., 'Liberals, Labour and Local Elections', in G. Peale and C. Cook, eds, *The Politics of Reappraisal, 1918–1938* (London, 1975), 166–88.
Crowther, M. A., *British Social Policy* (Basingstoke, 1988).

Daunton, M., *Wealth and Welfare: An Economic and Social History of Britain 1851–1951* (Oxford, 2007).

Davidson, R., and R. Lowe, 'Bureaucracy and Innovation in British Welfare Policy 1890–1945', in W. J. Mommsen, ed., *The Emergence of the Welfare State in Britain and Germany, 1850–1950* (London, 1981), 263–95.

Davies, B., *Social Needs and Resources in Local Services: A Study of Variations in Standards of Provision of Personal Social Services Between Local Authority Areas* (London, 1968).

Davies, S., and B. Morley, *County Borough Elections in England and Wales, 1919–1938*, i: *Barnsley – Bournemouth* (Aldershot and Brookfield, Vermont, 1999).

Davis, H., *The History of the Borough of Newport: From Swamp to Super-Town* (Newport, 1998).

Davis, J., 'Central Government and the Towns' in M. Daunton, ed., *The Cambridge Urban History of Britain*, iii: *1840–1950* (Cambridge, 2000), 261–86.

de Swaan, A., *In Care of the State: Health Care, Education and Welfare in Europe and the USA in the Modern Era* (Cambridge, 1990).

Digby, A., and N. Bosanquet, 'Doctors and Patients in an Era of National Health Insurance and Private Practice, 1913–1938', *Economic History Review*, 41:1 (1988), 74–94.

Dilks, D., *Neville Chamberlain*, i: *Pioneering and Reform, 1869–1929* (Cambridge, 1984).

Doyle, B., 'The Changing Functions of Urban Government', in M. Daunton, ed., *The Cambridge Urban History of Britain*, iii: *1840–1950* (Cambridge, 2000), 287–313.

Doyle, B., 'Competition and Cooperation in Hospital Provision in Middlesbrough, 1918–1948', *Medical History*, 51:3 (2007), 337–56.

Duprée, M., 'The Provision of Social Services' in M. Daunton, ed., *The Cambridge Urban History of Britain*, iii: *1840–1950* (Cambridge, 2000), 351–94.

Eckstein, H., *The English Health Service: Its Origins, Structure and Achievements* (Cambridge, Mass, 1958).

Eyler, J., 'Scarlet Fever and Confinement: The Edwardian Debate Over Isolation Hospitals', *Bulletin of the History of Medicine*, 61 (1987), 1–24.

Eyler, J., *Sir Arthur Newsholme and State Medicine 1885–1935* (Cambridge, 1997).

Feiling, K., *The Life of Neville Chamberlain* (Hamden, Conn, 1970, first published 1946).

Finlayson, G., *Citizen, State and Social Welfare in Britain, 1830–1990* (Oxford, 1994).

Foot, M., *Aneurin Bevan: A Biography*, 2 vols (London 1966 and 1975).

Foster, C., R. Jackman and M. Perlman, *Local Government Finance in a Unitary State* (London, 1980).
Fovargue, H. W., *Municipal Eastbourne, 1883–1933 – Selections From the Proceedings of the Town Council* (Eastbourne, 1933).
Fox, D. M., *Health Policies, Health Politics: The British and American Experience, 1911–1965* (Princeton, 1986).
Fraser, D., *The Evolution of the British Welfare State* (3rd edn, Basingstoke, 2003).
Frazer, W. M., *A History of English Public Health, 1834–1939* (London, 1950).
Garside, W. R., *British Unemployment, 1919–39* (Cambridge, 1990).
Gibbons, I. G., 'The Ministry of Health', *Journal of Public Administration*, 4:3 (1926), 243–66.
Gilbert, B., *Britain Since 1918* (1967; 2nd edn, London, 1980).
Gilbert, B. B., *British Social Policy 1914–1939* (London, 1970).
Gladstone, D., *The Twentieth-Century Welfare State* (Basingstoke, 1999).
Gorsky, M., J. Mohan and M. Powell, 'British Voluntary Hospitals, 1871–1938: The Geography of Provision and Utilization', *Journal of Historical Geography*, 25 (1999), 468–74.
Gorsky, M., and J. Mohan, 'London's Voluntary Hospitals in the Interwar Period', *Nonprofit and Voluntary Sector Quarterly*, 30:2 (2001), 247–75.
Gorsky, M., 'The Gloucestershire Extension of Medical Services Scheme: An Experiment in the Integration of Health Services in Britain Before the NHS', *Medical History*, 50:4 (2006), 491–512.
Gorsky, M. 'Public Health in Interwar England and Wales: Did it Fail?' *Dynamis*, 28 (2008), 175–98.
Gray, A., 'A Mixed Economy of Health Care: Britain's Health Service Sector in the Inter-War Period' in A. McGuire, P. Fenn and K. Mayhew, eds, *Providing Health Care: The Economics of Alternative Systems of Finance and Delivery* (Oxford, 1991), 233–60.
Grønlie, T., 'Norwegian General Hospitals, 1970–2002: County Ownership – an Interlude Between Welfare Localism and State Direction', *Medical History*, 50:2 (2006), 189–208.
Hansen, T., 'Transforming Needs into Expenditure Decisions', in K. Newton and F. Pinter, eds, *Urban Political Economy* (London, 1981), 27–47.
Hardy, A., *Health and Medicine in Britain Since 1860* (Basingstoke, 2001).
Harling, P., *The Modern British State: An Historical Introduction* (Cambridge, 2001).
Harris, B., *The Origins of the British Welfare State: Society, State and Social Welfare in England and Wales, 1800–1945* (Basingstoke, 2004).
Hastings, S., *The Hospital Services*, Fabian Research Series: 59 (London, 1941).

Hicks, J. R., and U. K. Hicks, 'Standards of Local Expenditure: A Problem of the Inequality of Incomes', *Occasional Papers*, National Institute of Economic and Social Research (Cambridge, 1943).
Hoggart, K., *Economy, Polity and Urban Public Expenditure* (Aldershot and Vermont, 1989).
Hodgkinson, R., *The Origins of the National Health Service* (London, 1967).
Hollingsworth, J. R., *A Political Economy of Medicine: Great Britain and the United States* (Baltimore, 1986).
Hollingsworth, J. R., and E. J. Hollingsworth, 'Public Organizations: The Behaviour of Hospitals in England and Wales' in E. James ed., *The Nonprofit Sector in International Perspective* (Oxford, 1990), 110–36.
Honigsbaum, F., *Health, Happiness and Security* (London, 1989).
Jenkins, S., *Accountable to None: The Tory Nationalization of Britain* (Harmondsworth, 1996)
Jones, K., *The Making of Social Policy in Britain: From the Poor Law to New Labour* (London, 2000).
Keith-Lucas, B., and P. G. Richards, *A History of Local Government in the Twentieth Century* (London, 1978).
King, D. N., 'Why do Local Authority Rate Poundages Differ?', *Public Administration*, 51 (1973), 165–73.
Klein, R., *The New Politics of the NHS: From Creation to Reinvention* (4th edn, Oxford, 2001)
Labour Party, *National Service for Health* (London, 1943).
Laski, H. J., I. Jennings, W. A. Robson and E. Halévy, *A Century of Municipal Progress* (London, 1935).
Laybourn, K., *Britain on the Breadline: A Social and Political History of Britain 1918–1939* (Stroud, 1998).
Le Grand, J., *The Strategy of Equality: Redistribution and the Social Services* (London, 1982).
Lee, R., 'Uneven Zenith: Towards a Geography of the High Period of Municipal Medicine in England and Wales', *Journal of Historical Geography* 14 (1988), 260–80.
Lester, A. M., 'William George Willoughby, MD, DPH, Medical Officer of Health to Eastbourne, 1894–1939', *Eastbourne Medical Gazette*, 3:1 (183) 20–2.
Levene, A., 'Between Less Eligibility and the NHS: The Changing Place of Poor Law Hospitals in England and Wales, 1929–39', *Twentieth Century British History*, 20:3 (2009), 322–45.
Levene, A., M. Powell and J. Stewart, 'Patterns of Municipal Health Expenditure in Interwar England and Wales', *Bulletin of the History of Medicine*, 78 (2004), 635–69.

Levene, A., M. Powell and J. Stewart, 'The Development of Municipal General Hospitals in English County Boroughs in the 1930s', *Medical History*, 50:1 (2006), 3–28.
Lewis, J., *The Politics of Motherhood: Child and Maternal Welfare in England, 1900–1939* (London, 1980).
Lewis, J., *What Price Community Medicine? The Philosophy, Practice and Politics of Public Health Since 1919* (Brighton, 1986).
Lipman, V. D., 'The Development of Areas and Boundary Changes 1888–1939', in C. H. Wilson, ed., *Essays on Local Government* (Oxford, 1948), 25–66.
Loudon, I., 'Some International Features of Maternal Mortality, 1880–1950', in V. A. Fildes, L. Marks and H. Marland, eds, *Women and Children First: International Maternal and Infant Welfare, 1870–1945* (London, 1992), 5–28.
Loughlin, M., M. David Gelfand and K. Young, eds, *Half a Century of Municipal Decline, 1935–1985* (London, 1985).
Lowe, R., and N. Rollings, 'Modernising Britain, 1957–64: A Classic Case of Centralisation and Fragmentation?' in R. A. W. Rhodes, ed., *Transforming British Government*, i: *Changing Institutions* (London, 2000), 99–118.
Mackintosh, J. M., *Trends in Opinion About the Public Health, 1901–51* (London, 1953).
Marks, L., *Metropolitan Maternity: Maternal and Infant Welfare in Early Twentieth-Century London* (Amsterdam, 1996).
Marshall, T. H., *Citizenship and Social Class* (London, 1950).
Menzies, F., 'Postwar British Medicine', *Medical Care*, 2:4 (1942), 337–46.
Midwinter, E., *The Development of Social Welfare in Britain* (Buckingham, 1994).
Millward, R., and F. Bell, 'Economic Factors in the Decline of Mortality in Late Nineteenth-Century Britain', *European Review of Economic History*, 2 (1998), 263–88.
Millward, R., 'Local Government Expenditure in Britain, 1870–1914: An Economic Analysis', *University of Manchester: Working Papers in Economic and Social History*, 27.
Mohan, J., *Planning, Markets and Hospitals* (London, 2002).
Mohan, J., 'Voluntarism, Municipalism and Welfare: The Geography of Hospital Utilization in England in 1938', *Transactions of the Institute of British Geographers*, 28 (2003), 56–74.
Morgan, K. O., *Consensus and Disunity: The Lloyd George Coalition Government, 1918–22* (Oxford, 1986).
Newcomer, M., *Central and Local Finance in Germany and England* (New York, 1937).

Newton, K., 'Central Government Grants, Territorial Justice and Local Democracy in Post-War Britain', in D. Ashford, ed., *Financing Urban Government in the Welfare State* (London, 1980), 97–118.

Oliver, F. R., and J. Stanyer, 'Some Aspects of the Financial Behaviour of County Boroughs', *Public Administration*, 47 (1969), 169–84.

Orwell, G., *The Road to Wigan Pier* (New Edn, London, 1989).

Overy, R., *The Morbid Age: Britain Between the Wars* (London, 2009).

Page, E., 'The Value of Local Autonomy', *Local Government Studies* 8:4 (1982), 21–42.

Page, E., *Localism and Centralism in Europe* (Oxford, 1991).

Page, E., and M. Goldsmith, 'Centre and Locality', in E. Page and M. Goldsmith, eds, *Central and Local Government Relations* (London: 1987), 1–11.

Pater, J. E., *The Making of the National Health Service* (London, 1981).

Peden, G., *British Economic and Social Policy: Lloyd George to Margaret Thatcher* (2nd edn, Hemel Hempstead, 1991).

Peretz, E., 'The Costs of Modern Motherhood to Low Income Families in Interwar Britain' in V. A. Fildes, L. Marks and H. Marland, eds, *Women and Children First: International Maternal and Infant Welfare, 1870–1945* (London, 1992), 257–80.

Peretz, E., 'Infant Welfare Between the Wars' in R. C. Whiting, ed., *Oxford: Studies in the History of a University Town Since 1800* (Manchester, 1993), 131–45.

Philo, C., 'Journey to Asylum: A Medical-Geographical Idea in Historical Context', *Journal of Historical Geography*, 21:2 (1995), 146–68.

Pickstone, J., *Medical and Industrial Society: A History of Hospital Development in Manchester and its Region, 1752–1946* (Manchester, 1985).

Pinker, R., *English Hospital Statistics 1861–1938* (London, 1966).

Powell, M., 'A Tale of Two Cities: A Critical Evaluation of the Geographic Provision of Health Care Before the NHS', *Public Administration*, 70 (Spring 1992), 67–80.

Powell, M., 'Hospital Provision Before the NHS: Territorial Justice or Inverse Care Law?', *Journal of Social Policy*, 21:2 (1992), 145–63.

Powell, M., 'Did Politics Matter? Municipal Health Expenditure in the 1930s', *Urban History*, 22:3 (1995), 360–79.

Powell, M., 'An Expanding Service: Municipal Acute Medicine in the 1930s', *Twentieth Century British History*, 8:3 (1997), 334–57.

Powell, M., 'In What Sense a National Health Service?', *Public Policy and Administration 13:3 (1998), 56–70.*

Powell, M., and G. Boyne, 'The Spatial Strategy of Equality and the Spatial Division of Welfare', *Social Policy and Administration* (2001), 181–94.

Powell, M., 'What was Wales? Towards a Contextual Approach to Medical History' in P. Michael and C. Webster, eds, *Health and Society in Twentieth-Century Wales* (Cardiff, 2007), 216–39.
Preston, B. T., 'Rich Town, Poor Town: The Distribution of Rate-Bourne Spending Levels in the Edwardian City System', *Transactions of the Institute of British Geographers*, New Series, 10 (1985), 77–94.
Pugh, M., '*We Danced All Night': A Social History of Britain Between the Wars* (London, 2008).
Rhodes, E. H., 'Personality in Public Administration', *Journal of Public Administration*, 8:3 (1930), 250–2.
Robson, W., *The Development of Local Government* (rev. edn, London, 1948).
Robson, W. A., 'Labour and Local Government', *Political Quarterly* 24:1 (1953), 39–53
Savage, M., 'Rise of the Labour Party in Local Perspective', *Journal of Regional and Local Studies*, 10:1 (1990), 1–15.
Self, R., *Neville Chamberlain: A Biography* (Aldershot, 2006).
Sharpe, L. J., and K. Newton, *Does Politics Matter? The Determinants of Public Policy* (Oxford, 1984).
Sheard, S., 'Reluctant Providers? The Politics and Ideology of Municipal Hospital Finance 1870–1914' in M. Gorsky and S. Sheard, eds, *Financing Medicine: The British Experience Since 1750* (London, 2006), 112–29.
Smith, F. B., *The Retreat of Tuberculosis 1850–1950* (London, 1988).
Stevenson, J., *English Social History 1914–45* (Harmondsworth, 1984).
Stewart, J., 'Socialist Proposals for Health Reform in Inter-War Britain: The Case of Somerville Hastings', *Medical History*, 39:3 (1995), 338–57.
Stewart, J., '"For a Healthy London": The Socialist Medical Association and the London County Council in the 1930s', *Medical History*, 41:4 (1997), 417–36.
Stewart, J., *The Battle for Health: A Political History of the Socialist Medical Association, 1930–51* (Aldershot, 1999).
Stewart, J., '"The Finest Municipal Hospital Service in the World"?: Contemporary Perceptions of the London County Council's Hospital Provision, 1929–1939', *Urban History*, 32:2 (2005), 327–44.
Stewart, J., 'The Mixed Economy of Welfare in Historical Context', in M. Powell, ed., *Understanding the Mixed Economy of Welfare* (Bristol, 2007).
Surtees, J., *The Princess Alice and Other Eastbourne Hospitals* (Eastbourne, 1994).
Tanner, D., 'The Pattern of Labour Politics, 1918–1939' in D. Tanner, C. Williams and D. Hopkin, eds, *The Labour Party in Wales, 1900–2000* (Cardiff, 2000), 114–35.
Tanner, D., 'Labour and its Membership' in D. Tanner, P. Thane and N. Tiratsoo, eds, *Labour's First Century* (Cambridge, 2000), 248–80.

Taylor, A. J. P., *English History 1914–1945* (Harmondsworth, 1970).
Thane, P., *Foundations of the Welfare State* (2nd edn, Harlow, 1996).
Thompson, S., 'Unemployment, Poverty and Women's Health in Inter-war Wales', in P. Michael and C. Webster, eds, *Health and Society in Twentieth Century Wales* (Cardiff, 2006), 98–122.
Thorpe, A., *Britain in the 1930s* (Oxford, 1992).
Timmins, N., *The Five Giants: A Biography of the Welfare State* (revised edn. London, 2001).
Titmuss, R., *Problems of Social Policy* (London, 1950).
Wallace, D. E., *Reports of Investigations into the Industrial Conditions in Certain Depressed Areas, Part II, Durham and Teesside* (London, 1934).
Ward, S. V., 'Implementation Versus Planmaking: The Example of List Q and the Depressed Areas 1922–39', *Planning Perspectives*, 1 (1986), 3–26.
Ward, S. V., *The Geography of Interwar Britain: The State and Uneven Development* (London, 1988).
Warren, J. H., *The English Local Government System* (London, 1946).
Watts, J., and D. Nannestad, *The First Fifty Years – Half a Century of Labour Rule in Barnsley* (Barnsley, 1983).
Webster, C., 'Healthy or Hungry Thirties?', *History Workshop Journal*, 8 (1982), 110–29.
Webster, C., 'Health, Welfare and Unemployment During the Depression', *Past and Present*, 109 (1985), 204–30.
Webster, C., *The Health Services Since the War*, i: *Problems of Health Care – The National Health Service Before 1957* (London, 1988).
Webster, C., 'Labour and the Origins of the National Health Service', in N. Rupke, ed., *Science Politics and the Public Good* (Basingstoke, 1988), 184–202.
Webster, C., 'Conflict and Consensus: Explaining the British Health Service', *Twentieth Century British History*, 1:2 (1990), 115–51.
Welshman, J., *Municipal Medicine: Public Health in Twentieth Century Britain* (Bern, 2000).
White, J., 'From Herbert Morrison to Command and Control: The Decline of Local Democracy and its Effect on Public Services', *History Workshop Journal*, 59:1 (2005), 73–82.
Whitehead, M., *National Health Success* (London, 1988).
Williams, M., '"The Growing Toll of Motherhood": Maternal Mortality in Wales', in P. Michael and C. Webster, eds, *Health and Society in Twentieth Century Wales* (Cardiff, 2006), 123–42.
Willis, T., 'The Bradford Municipal Hospital Experiment of 1920' in M. Gorsky and S. Sheard, eds, *Financing Medicine: The British Experience Since 1750* (London, 2006), 130–44.

Wilson, D., and C. Game, *Local Government in the United Kingdom* (Basingstoke, 2002).
Wilson, N., *Public Health Services* (London, 1938).
Wilson, N., *Municipal Health Services* (London, 1946).
Worboys, M., 'The Sanatorium Treatment for Consumption in Britain 1890–1914', in J. Pickstone, ed., *Medical Innovations in Historical Perspective* (Basingstoke, 1992), 47–71.
Worley, M., *Labour Inside the Gate: A History of the British Labour Party Between the Wars* (London, 2005).

Internet Sources

Dictionary of National Biography.

Sheard, S., 'Mixed Motives: Improving the Health of Seamen in Liverpool 1875–1939', <http://phoenixtn.net/publication/evora/papersOriginal/ MixedMotivesHealthofSeamen.doc> accessed 9 March 2010.
Szreter, S., 'A Central Role for Local Government? The Example of Late Victorian Britain', *History and Policy* [online journal] (2002). http://www.historyandpolicy.org/papers/policy-paper-01.html
White, J., 'From Herbert Morrison to Command and Control: The Decline of Local Democracy' *History and Policy* [online journal] (2004), < http://www.historyandpolicy.org/papers/policy-paper-18.html> (accessed 17 July 2009).

Unpublished Work

Beach, A. L., 'The Labour Party and the Idea of Citizenship, c. 1931–1951', PhD thesis, University of London, 1996.
Bradbury, J. P., 'The 1929 Local Government Act: The Formulation and Implementation of Poor Law (Health Care) and Exchequer Grants Reform for England and Wales (Outside London)', PhD thesis, University of Bristol, 1991.

Cutts, V., 'Health During the Inter-War Period in the Mining Town of Barnsley', dissertation, Leeds University, 1981 [degree unspecified].
Lindley, T., 'The Party Machine: A Study of Barnsley Labour Party and its Leaders, 1918–1945', dissertation for the Social Studies Diploma, Ruskin College, 1978.
Neville, J., 'Explaining Variations in Municipal Hospital Provision in the 1930s: A Study of Councils in the Far South West', PhD thesis, University of Exeter, 2010.
Rowett, J., 'The Labour Party and Local Government: Theory and Practice in the Interwar Years', DPhil thesis, University of Oxford, 1979.
Stacey, S. R., 'The Ministry of Health, 1919–29: Ideas and Practice in a Government Department', DPhil thesis, University of Oxford, 1984.
Wilson, R., 'The Economy, Housing and Health in West Hartlepool, 1919–1939', MPhil thesis, University of Teesside, no date.

Index

Tables and Figures are indicated by page numbers in *italics*.

Studies in the History of Medicine

Edited by Charles Webster, All Souls College, Oxford

Studies in the History of Medicine provides an outlet for academic monographs devoted to both the social and the intellectual dimensions of the history of medicine. No limitations are imposed with respect to period or place, providing the approach adopted is analytical and historical. The series encourages investigations relating to previously neglected aspects of medicine and health care such as the history of nursing or other occupations associated with health care, case studies of particular disease and illness phenomena, health care in colonial and postcolonial settings, or indeed complementary medicine, dentistry or veterinary medicine. The monographs inevitably evaluate the impact of modern high-technology medicine, but they also give appropriate weight to health care as it relates to the elderly, the mentally ill or other vulnerable social groups. Except in special circumstances the series will not include general biographies, histories of individual institutions and organisations, or studies of parochial interest. The monographs included in this series reflect the leading edge of research in the now well-established and still expanding field of medical history.

Vol. 1 John Welshman. Municipal Medicine: Public Health in Twentieth-Century Britain. 2000. 339 pp.
ISBN 3-906766-40-3 / US-ISBN 0-8204-5327-7

Vol. 2 Jacqueline Jenkinson. Scotland's Health 1919–1948. 2002. 506 pp.
ISBN 3-906768-34-1 / US-ISBN 0-8204-5622-5

Vol. 3 Charles Webster. The Great Instauration: Science, Medicine and Reform 1626–1660. 2002. 670 pp.
ISBN 3-906768-37-6 / US-ISBN 0-8204-5616-0

Vol. 4 Alysa Levene, Martin Powell, John Stewart and Becky Taylor. Cradle to Grave: Municipal Medicine in Interwar England and Wales. 2011. 270 pp.
ISBN 978-3-03910-904-3

Vol. 5 Anne Digby. Diversity and Division in Medicine: Health care in South Africa from the 1800s. 2006. 504 pp.
ISBN 3-03910-715-1 / US-ISBN 0-8204-7978-0

www.ingramcontent.com/pod-product-compliance
Ingram Content Group UK Ltd.
Pitfield, Milton Keynes, MK11 3LW, UK
UKHW020200290926
15471UKWH00005B/983